T0202086

# WOMEN,
# HEALTHCARE,
# AND
# VIOLENCE
# IN
# PAKISTAN

# WOMEN, HEALTHCARE, AND VIOLENCE IN PAKISTAN

SARA RIZVI JAFREE

THE **PLATINUM** SERIES

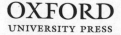

OXFORD
UNIVERSITY PRESS

# OXFORD
UNIVERSITY PRESS

Oxford University Press is a department of the University of Oxford.
It furthers the University's objective of excellence in research, scholarship,
and education by publishing worldwide. Oxford is a registered trade mark of
Oxford University Press in the UK and in certain other countries

Published in Pakistan by
Ameena Saiyid, Oxford University Press
No.38, Sector 15, Korangi Industrial Area,
PO Box 8214, Karachi-74900, Pakistan

ISBN 978-0-19-940606-7

Printed on 80gsm Local Offset Paper

Printed by Mas Printers, Karachi

## Dedication

For my grandfathers, Dada Baba (1918–90) and Nana (1924–2014), and my father-in-law and father, Abu and Baba. They have been the best protectors, guides, and role models a daughter could wish for.

# Contents

# Acknowledgements

In the course of researching organizational culture and its association with error-reporting in the hospitals of Pakistan, I began discussing my recurrent findings across designations and hospitals with my grandmother and aunt. They encouraged me to work on this book notwithstanding the widely prevalent tendency of researchers and working women to shy away from disclosing sensitive details about workplace violence in a country with a culture that severely inhibits this. I have been surrounded and blessed with incredible mothers, my grandmothers Syeda Laila Rezvi and Syeda Sikander Rezvi, and my aunts and mother, Rehana Asad, Khadija Mohib, Rabia Shah, and Zehra Shah, who have always encouraged me to fearlessly speak my mind.

My entry into the world of research would not have been possible without the support and generosity of the late Professor Dr Muhammad Hafeez. He was a remarkable guide and mentor for every individual who had the good fortune to cross his path. His patriotism was contagious and most of his students, including myself, have him to thank for our commitment to the community and nation in all we do, whether working on projects or making life-altering decisions. I owe my understanding of the rigorous processes of research and data analysis to my Professors Drs Zakria Zakar and Rubeena Ashraf Zakar. There is no doubt in my mind that without their support I would still be a struggling PhD scholar, incapable of converting my data into transmittable knowledge and of making this book a reality. Communication skills when interviewing people is also something that I have learnt from them.

I must also thank my FCCU family: My Dean, Dr General Noel Khokhar, and Drs Julie Flowerday, Rukhsana Zia, and Sufian Aslam, along with so many others who have always been available for advice, guidance, and encouragement. I must also express my gratitude to Drs Eileen Lake and Linda Aiken in guiding my use of internationally accepted methods of research. I am also greatly indebted to all the women practitioner respondents who participated in the survey and all the male and female practitioners who agreed to be interviewed for this study. I owe all the findings set out here to them. There are many other senior scholars and academicians to whom I owe a debt of gratitude for their constant encouragement, particularly when I felt I could not manage this project alone, including Mrs Nasreen Shah, Dr Riffat Munawar, Dr Ahmad Khalil, and Mrs Amber Tariq.

This book could not have materialized without the assistance of my amazing team of researchers to whom I owe a deep debt of gratitude for their tireless and ceaseless hard work and loyalty. They were always there to support me with permissions and gatekeeping issues, coordination of meetings with practitioners, pilot-testing, survey, data collection, and extended qualitative interviews. This includes Uroosa Yousaf, Yumna Fiaz, Khadija Naeem, Aasma Fiaz, Begum Najma, and Dr Zakia Hussain. Two other research assistants, Barrister Mohammad Ali and Aneeq Sarwar, provided immense support in the interviews of male healthcare practitioners and senior health administrators.

Invaluable support was provided by the gatekeepers and contact points, including practitioners and administrators, without whom I would have been unable to gain official permission for research and repeated entry for meetings. These include Drs Nafeesah Fatima, Mahwish Naz, Madiha Ilyas, Zunaira Shafique, Qurut-ul-Ain, Sisters Nasira Iqbal and Tauseef Khurshid, Dr Hafiz Asim, Zakia Qazafi, Supervisors Asia Iqbal, Asmat Shahid, Maryam Naseer, Naila Farid, and Nusrat Ramzan. Thanks are also due to my friends and colleagues, trained clinical psychologists, Aaleen Zaryab and Amna Khawar, for agreeing to share their time to counsel women practitioner victims. Experienced healthcare practitioners who have been generous in their guidance and discussion of findings include Drs Professor Hamid Ali, Professor Syed Sibtul Hasnain, Mujtaba Nadir Shah, Aliya Rani Sial, Shakeela Sheikh, and Shahmila Ijaz Munir. I also thank Barrister Mohammad Nabeel Khan Dahir for helping out with legal issues and clarifications. Thanks to Murtaza Hasnain, Mudasir Mustafa, and Alina Alam for accurate proofreading of the manuscript. I must add that Dr Anwar Mughal, Mustafa Hasnain, and Snowber Humayoun were of great help in all my struggles and queries relating to IT and SPSS.

My gratitude to my brothers Amaar Hyder and Hammad Abbas and their wives for their continuing support; they will always remain my home away from home. My beloved sisters Ambareen, Sehba, Nouchine, and Saira have been constant sources of inspiration. They have always been hard working women, who in their quiet ways continue to inspire me on how to balance home and work life. I have lost an integral member of my household this year, my mother-in-law. It is difficult to explain to some people in Punjab that the loss of a mother-in-law does not mean the usurpation of her role, but rather of a circle being broken forever. I am grateful for the lessons she taught me during her lifetime and her prayers from heaven, upon which I depend for the protection of my husband and children. Finally, my husband, Baqir, and my daughters, Aliza and Alina, deserve my greatest gratitude. They are the greatest gifts God has given me and inspire me daily to become a better person and to work harder.

Sara Rizvi Jafree
20 July 2017

# Introduction

The region known as India in the past and currently as South Asia extends from Burma to Afghanistan and includes Pakistan. The 1.7 billion people belonging to this region comprise eight different nationalities, speak over 33 languages, and follow six religions which are Hinduism, Islam, Christianity, Jainism, Buddhism, and Sikhism. Notwithstanding an awareness of the economic necessity of female work participation and the monetary requirement for their well-being, to minimize organizational and national costs, workplace violence remains a very consistent human rights violation. Estimates suggest that every third woman suffers from workplace violence across the globe (OXFAM 2012), with the highest rates of violence being faced by women working in the health sector (Di Martino 2002). Pakistani media reports and scholarship both hint at a high incidence of workplace violence against women practitioners but due to an absence of formal monitoring by the state, there is no hard data about the actual prevalence. Scholarship and funding has de-emphasized workplace violence against women and placed domestic violence at the forefront of research and policy initiatives (Wiskow 2003). Besides, feminization of poverty and the need to raise the level of labour participation of women has sidelined initiatives to secure the safety and protection of women in the workforce.

Nearly three-fourths of the Pakistani population lives below the poverty line, of which a majority are women, principally due to illiteracy, meagre ownership of resources, and unemployment (Hassan & Farooq 2015). Of the 26 per cent of women in Pakistan who are participating in the labour force, a majority are engaged in semi-skilled jobs, low status work, and inferior pay (World Economic Forum, 2015). This is especially so for nurses and lady healthcare workers who comprise a majority of the women healthcare practitioners in the country. An approximate total of 976,562 women healthcare practitioners, including doctors, nurses, and lady healthcare workers, are front line specialists in Pakistan. They shoulder a heavy burden in ensuring patient safety in the public sector hospitals used by 30 per cent of the population (Akbari et al., 2009), and also play an exclusive role in ensuring the well-being of women and children. When women healthcare practitioners are provided a safe work environment, their care provision and role delivery is favourable, thus ensuring patient health and mortality (McNamara 2010). However, women workers in the health sector face disincentives to work and perform optimally due to the constant threat of violence they face. Some estimates predict that over 90 per cent of women practitioners face violence daily at the workplace in some form or the other in developing regions (American Psychiatric Nurses Association Position Statement 2008). The determinants of verbal and physical violence, professional bullying, and sexual abuse comprises deep-rooted socio-cultural prejudices and organizational injustices which are entwined in the fabric of a community's traditions and socio-structural systems.

After six years of research on the organizational culture of the public healthcare sector in Pakistan, I found that the most neglected area related to workplace violence faced by women practitioners. I was therefore anxious to remedy this, particularly in view of the fact that Pakistani society, as many others, resents women's revelation of instances of abuse. However, I was also concerned about what impact my intrusion into this area would have. My problems and the barriers I faced in terms of data collection will be discussed in detail in the book. This work attempts to understand and map the myriad forms of and reasons for the violence faced by women practitioners in their respective communities and workplaces. The safety of women healthcare practitioners needs to be ensured through the enactment of reformative laws, correction of religious representation, and improvement in state and health sector policies. These are possible through a growth in academic scholarship in this significant area.

Women in South Asia have been restricted for centuries to domestic and reproductive roles (Solotaroff & Pande 2014). When they have been employed for work outside the home, due to financial and social necessity, they have been subjected to defamation and violence. The earliest historical records from South Asia list homeopathy and herbal medicine such as Ayurveda[1] and Unani[2] as the principal sources of healing. In the past, the services of women with a passion for healing, or the inherited knowledge from their ancestors, were utilized in the absence of male healers, and particularly for the treatment of female patients (Ehrenreich 2010). However, they were largely classified as midwife or helper and considered much inferior to the traditional male healers (Chaudhury & Rafei 2001). Thus, for many centuries, women did provide healing but without degrees, gratitude, and opportunities for knowledge exchange. Although history acknowledges that women healers were sometimes referred to as 'wise women', it also confirms that they were more commonly labelled as 'witches' or 'charlatans'. It was the latter labels that encouraged violence and homicide against traditional women healers and also vindicated their perpetrators. Many traditional women healers provided natural remedies for birth spacing, the reproductive health of mothers, and immunization of children. However, the conservative communities of the past regarded such women healers as perilous intercessors and did not pass up opportunities of victimization, especially in the face of maternal and child health complications or mortality. Although laws regulating the practice of traditional medicine exist, no edicts in the past or present have prevented violence against traditional women healers (World Health Organization 2001).

The first historical evidence from the Indian subcontinent about the formal inclusion of women as healthcare providers in the workforce was during the rule of King Asoka.[3] During Asoka's reign, between 268 to 232 BCE, state resources were allocated to the cultivation of medical herbs and the establishment of health dispensaries throughout the kingdom (Dhammika 1993). Asoka's central political philosophy, inspired by Buddhist principles (Friedlander 2009), was to cater to the health needs of everyone, specifically of vulnerable groups such as women and children, the elderly, and even animals. Eventually, Buddhist nuns were also recruited to fill the gender gap in the health workforce (Seneviratna 1995). The nuns cared for the nutrition and healing of the sick and the infirm, and in particular were the principal care providers for women (Ohnuma 2006). They used a combination of Ayurveda and mystical practices to treat the community and were responsible for imparting knowledge about healing and care provision to younger nuns (Agarwal & Kapil 2016).

The medicine men and physicians of Asoka's time followed the Charaka medical philosophies and care plans.[4] The outline of medical procedures, the description of hospitals, and the detailed classification of drugs were a legacy of Charaka (Murlidhar & Byadgi 2011; Valiathan 2003). Charaka's guidelines for the physician and hospital administration were documented exclusively for men, as then only men occupied these positions. No allowance was made for female care providers except as inferior assistants required for female patients and for lowly nursing duties. Charaka's medical philosophy still prevails, keeping the medical profession within the masculine domain, and keeping development decisions, research, and governance away from the purview of women practitioners.

Women nurses, as we know them today, are a legacy of the Christian Crimean wars, fought from 1853 to 1856. When Florence Nightingale declared her intention to become a nurse, her family went into a state of shock and her father refused to grant her permission to do so (Cohen 1984). In Europe, for the daughters of upper class families, it was impossible to even consider a profession in nursing. The popularity and honour surrounding Nightingale was not shared by the vast majority of other nurses at the time. The difficulties for other women nurses can best be illustrated through the life story of Mary Seacole, who was refused an interview for military nursing in the Crimean War due to her Jamaican ethnicity. She used her personal funds to make the journey to the war zone and also to pay for the supplies used for wounded soldiers. She returned from Crimea destitute and ailing, and received no fame for her efforts (Klainberg 2010). It is clear that race and socio-economic belonging has a very strong linkage with the status and safety of women healthcare practitioners.

It is possible that Nightingale received acknowledgement for her services due to her upper class background. Even today, the research for this book indicates, which is supported by the works of other scholars, that class plays a major role in the victimization of women practitioners, with the lower classes suffering the greatest neglect, abuse, and aggression at the workplace. Many of the soldiers of the Crimean War, who were nursed by Seacole and other women from lower class backgrounds, are known to have been the originators of the tales of the romantic relationships between patients and nurses. Passionate songs and poetry, that may originally have been harmlessly dedicated to lower class nurses, have over time led to the sexual objectification of women nurses and has undermined their professional status. Perceiving women nurses as sexual objects, as opposed to trained practitioners, is recognized as having precipitated violence against women practitioners at the workplace.

Nightingale in the mid-nineteenth century aggressively encouraged women to become nurses rather than doctors. She advocated that women only made 'third-rate doctors' and it is possibly this belief of hers which helped to project a lower status for women doctors (Smith 1951). It is known that other pioneering nurses strongly decried women joining the medical profession in order to promote the professional status of nursing. This however had the effect of damaging the status of both the professions. Patriarchal societies, as in South Asia, have effectively used women icons like Florence Nightingale to feminize the nursing profession and encourage the public belief that women as doctors are inferior to men. The result has been that women are ineffective professionals, not worthy of the title 'doctor' and can have little expectation of high status and a positive identity. This combination of inferior labels, borne by both women nurses and women doctors, has led to their increased victimization in the region (Crowther 2001). The findings of this study, as reported in Chapter 7, confirm that the current competition and jealousy between women nurses and doctors has weakened gender solidarity and the mobilization for advancement and security.

The British colonizers of India preferred to bring their own nurses from Great Britain and it was these few élite nurses who remained at the top of the nursing hierarchy with benefits of higher status, compensation, and safety (Wilkinson 1958). In the twentieth century, missionaries in India began training indigenous nurses to serve the local population in need of medical care. The indigenous Indian nurses had comparatively inferior contracts and worked in disadvantaged conditions. As it was unthinkable for Muslim women to work out of their homes, nearly all the first group of nurses in South Asia were lower class Christian converts, Hindus, and destitute women in need of a livelihood, such as widows, divorcees, and orphans. Though nursing in India was established under the aegis of colonial rule, the rigid hierarchies that are evident today within the nursing and medical professions are also a legacy of the British. The 'white' nurses trained in England or of Anglo-Indian descent were retained for the colonial rulers and the upper class and the 'brown' native nurses deployed for the local population. The status demarcation between white lady nurses and the brown 'dirty' nurses created an environment which precipitated violence against the growing majority of the latter.

Indigenous nurses working for ordinary Indians were likened to lower caste prostitutes (Chew 2002). They rapidly emerged as an oppressed group, who commonly faced both horizontal violence from co-workers and general violence from the wider public. Not only were female nurses excluded from professional training but were considered inferior practitioners given their family responsibilities and childbearing. There are accounts of rape by British officers and local men, and this was the principal reason why only lower class women, desperate for a livelihood, entered the healthcare profession. Restricted social entry of lower class women nurses meant that the social perception and understanding of the nursing profession became synonymous with violence. Over time, as more nurses from the lower classes entered the profession, they began to experience re-victimization given their inability to report violence and seek accountability. This period served as a building block for the general social belief in the subcontinent that nursing was an inferior profession suitable for women alone. Nursing schools were opened as women's institutes, with women doctors subsequently entering medical schools, but in much smaller numbers (Forbes 1994).

Unfortunately, women doctors inherited the inferior labels attached to women nurses rather than inheriting the comparatively superior status of their male counterparts. It is clear that gender plays a powerful role in allocating an inferior status ascribed for women doctors rather than the achievement of the status they deserve on the strength of their training and merit. The result has been that women doctors received virtually no opportunities for professional advancement in comparison to their male counterparts. Initially, women in India were sucked into the healthcare workforce for one reason alone: to serve secluded women patients. In this way, their professional status was compromised as subservient members of the team limited to gynaecological and obstetric services (Nair & Healey 2006). The first female British doctor to practice in India, Dr Edith Pechey, helped develop the Dufferin Fund[5] in 1885, which was aimed at providing western healthcare to indigenous Indian women in zenana[6] hospitals (Burton 1996). In another two years over 150 women were enrolled in programmes to become not women doctors but 'hospital assistants'. Although most research indicates that these women were heroic front runners for women's empowerment, the truth is that they were vulnerable women who were very underpaid and made to deliver unskilled care. It is these 'hospital assistants' who faced violence from patients and supervisors given their low status, minimal training, and low-class social background. This kept their status low in the eyes of the public and also set the stage for the way in which indigenous women doctors would be regarded in the future.

One way for the colonial rulers to uproot traditional authority after 1830 was by sacrificing the cause of gender equality. In their bid to establish Western systems of education and law, the 'stick' was used to inaugurate healthcare centres and medical institutes; the 'carrot' that was offered was the retention of familiar male hierarchies and promoting male healthcare leaders and doctors. The difficulty in gaining admission to medical schools and inflexible licensing restrictions prevented women from practising medicine during this period (Witz 2001). Women doctors received accreditation very slowly, with some receiving only licensing documents and not university degrees (Crowther 2001). Notwithstanding extended training and passing examinations in medicine and surgery, the colonial authorities awarded qualified women with the lowly designation of 'hospital assistants'. There were certain regions where the governors did not recognize women doctors, making it difficult for them to practise, receive training, and acquire know-how from experienced male doctors. Here, imperialism, professional marginalization, and feminism combined to play a role in precipitating and sustaining violence against women healthcare practitioners of South Asia.

The celebrated Dufferin Fund was strictly intended for upper class élite Indian women. The discriminatory nature of resource allocation was made evident when funds were revoked for Dr Haimavati Sen's Imambargah Hospital by the Lieutenant Governor of Bengal (Sehrawat 2013). Dr Sen was treating lower class Indian women but, given a lack of finances she used to serve as an assistant to male surgeons in order to earn money and help her patients. It was not uncommon for many women doctors at this time to serve as assistants to male doctors or even worse, not have a licence to practise at all, thus depriving the public of life-saving services. Early resistance by male medical heads and hospital staff permitting women to practise and improve male medical models with care models and nursing plans was a patriarchal effort to retain control over the profession. Many argue that the limited training and professional autonomy provided to women doctors is a legacy of colonial rule.

The cultural tradition of purdah and the stereotyping of a virtuous Asian woman forced women to cover their faces in the presence of men and restricted them from communicating with men in the hospital regime. One of the principal reasons why women doctors in colonial India were unable to achieve high status was because of the constraining effect of purdah (Burton 1996). Even in zenana hospitals, women doctors had to interact with male populations (such as instructors, co-workers, ward assistants, compounders, and family attendants), and this created a negative impression. They stopped being likened to the 'gentle ladies' of the past and instead were labelled as polluted women; thus increasing their vulnerability to various forms of social exclusion and abuse. In addition, the material symbols that were expected to secure professional honour for women, including starched nursing uniforms, surgical scrubs, and doctor coats, were rejected by the public. Identification of the status of women practitioners was built through recognition of gender and the female form. Unfortunately, sexual objectification of women practitioners became more salient than the professional respect expected to be afforded by props such as uniforms and medical equipment (Kelly et al. 2012).

It is true that medical work for women has become unsexed in some modern industrial societies but this is not the case in South Asia. Women doctors and nurses have been, and still are, performing gendered work, which is considered to be of lower status and causes the female worker to become more vulnerable to violence. As professional status and violence have an intimate relationship, it is important to discuss elements that have contributed to the deterioration of the professional woman doctor. One of the reasons is that women doctors have been recruited to maintain the reproductive health of other women. Similar to their female clients, women doctors have also been oppressed, and in addition deprived of professional independence and autonomy. This can best be illustrated through the life of the first Indian woman doctor, Anandabai Joshee (Dall 1888). Encouraged by her husband and driven by the tragic death of her newly born son, Joshee overcame social hurdles and taboos to study medicine in 1886 from the Woman's Medical College of Pennsylvania. Although an iconic forerunner for other women in the region, she was also a significant role model for upholding regressive cultural norms.

She met with severe opposition from her relatives in her quest to travel to the US for medical studies, but instead of responding with resentment, she defended her critics with understanding and acceptance (Kosambi 1996). She anticipated that she would be victimized and excommunicated by her own people. One may call this attitude fatalism, blame acceptance, and victim ownership, but it is clear that Joshee set the stage for women doctors accepting their fate as social rebels who had to inevitably accept violence as a part of their job profile. On her return from the US, orthodox Hindu priests and other community members, including her family, accepted her but with contradictory labels of being an outsider and a rebel. This was nothing foreign to Joshee, who had been pelted with stones during her attempt to acquire secondary education in India. Rather than developing a sense of animosity and bitterness against her people, she embraced guilt and tolerance. During her short life, Joshee was known to staunchly uphold religious rites and cultural customs that went contrary to the concept of gender protection. Notwithstanding her exposure to knowledge and science, she ardently upheld the laws of Manu, which made it a sacred duty for wives to undergo all manner of hardship till death to satisfy their husbands. She gave equal importance to cooking and gardening and upheld marital customs which subordinated the wife, such as eating after serving her husband.

Not only did she give priority to her husband's well-being over her professional obligations but she even supported his view that child marriage had social advantages. Joshee's prolonged and painful suffering from tuberculosis, which led to her untimely death, was a remarkable display of uncomplaining serenity. This is possibly because Joshee accepted her death as a penance for straying from her primary duties outlined by religious and social covenants. It cannot be argued that her purpose in life was not to elevate the status of Indian women but her acceptance of social inequality against herself made it difficult for future women doctors to overcome rigid socio-professional stereotypes. The compromise that women doctors make with violence today may have its roots in the legacy of pioneering women like Joshee.

The social disapproval of independent decision-making by women from ancient times to the present day is demonstrated through societal disapproval of women's participation in the workforce. South Asian community leaders have nurtured the fear that an increase in women's work participation will pose a threat to the institution of marriage, joint families, and reproduction. It is believed that working women will compromise on their role as housewives, caring for their in-laws, and unquestioningly accepting the rulings of the male heads of the household. The danger with working women is that they would become rebellious and seek to make their own life decisions, such as choosing their spouse, demanding symmetrical household responsibilities, opting for divorce, and deciding how many children they wish to have. This is a risk which Muslim and other South Asian men have not wanted to take.

Marsha Norman confirms that the domestic role allocations for women are not just confined to developing and Muslim countries but are also true of the Western world (Spencer 1989). She argues that historically women have been used primarily to perform the role of 'cleaners' in times of sickness, death, and war. The standard social expectation from women is that they should keep their homes clean. Consequently, when a woman dares to join the workforce, the social expectation is that she will continue to fulfil the roles she has hitherto been performing within her home, such as care provision, emotional support, and blame acceptance. Even as trained care providers in the modern world, historical expectations of women's gendered roles affords them a lower status. In comparison to their male counterparts, women practitioners are still principally perceived as cleaners rather than as professionals.

The problem with Muslim countries is that frequently gender inequality issues are deterministically blamed on regressive Islamic interpretations and patriarchal dominance. Interestingly, nursing and medical services provided by women were legitimized and approved by the Prophet of Islam, Muhammad (PBUH) (Mebrouk 2008). There were some very important women companions of the Prophet who were given permission to participate in out-of-home healthcare services and were accorded high status for their contribution in the health workforce (Glubb 1963). This happened when the Prophet made the provision for nursing care an integral subpart of the Muslim army. Aisha bint Abu Bakr, Umme-e-Salim, and Umm-e-Salit were extremely proficient in nursing the wounded during times of war and in times of peace (Kelen 1977). The Prophet encouraged medical camps for patients and training camps for women interested in providing nursing and surgical services for the community. He also made it compulsory for all sects, races, and genders to be provided care and medical services without bias. Prominent women companions[7] were renowned for their skills in medicine and surgery, and were singled out by the Prophet as community leaders who were performing a sacred duty by saving lives. It was not possible for these women to be celebrated for their healing skills without some form of a systematic learning process, instruction, organization, and teamwork, which is precisely what contemporary medical and nursing schools are intended to do. Other women companions[8] used to stand guard at the rear end of the battlefield and pass arrows and supplies to male soldiers. They were known to contribute tactical assistance and even assist in fighting battles and burying the dead, in the event a shortage of male workers or soldiers occurred. It is evident that the modern interpretation of forced and rigid gender segregation in Islam, imposed by the Saudi government and other Muslim nations like Pakistan, upon education, employment, and public participation, has little authentic basis in Islam.

Prophet Muhammad's beloved daughter, Hazrat Fatima, was highly esteemed by him and called the leader of all Muslim women (Shariati 2014). Her actions and behaviour in relation to work participation outside of home have unfortunately not been widely known or understood by the Muslim community, and especially not in Pakistan. Hazrat Fatima performed nursing duties for her father and Muslim soldiers when they fought defensive battles in the early years of Islam (Kashani-Sabet 2005) and was referred to as 'mother' by the Prophet for her services. She was a prominent instructor for the interpretation of Quranic verses even for the companions and followers of the Prophet who were not her blood relatives, such as Hazrat Salman Farsi (Ordoni 2014). This demonstrates that Muslim women are permitted to seek knowledge from and impart it to men who are not their blood relatives. Most historical records confirm that Hazrat Fatima rushed to Uhud and nursed her father's wounds on the battlefield (Margoliouth & Muḥammad 1939). It is clear that she was following the soldiers in a logistical tent not far away in order to be available for nursing duties, and apparently this was part of the strategic plan. Public speeches and social counsel is not forbidden to women. Hazrat Fatima spoke publicly and served as a trusted counsellor on social issues relating to the home, religious law, and work participation. She, along with other woman companions, such as Umm-e Sulaim bint Malhan from the Ansar tribe, was known to undertake nursing responsibilities in battles even when pregnant. Inductively, the general disapproval of married women in Muslim societies pursuing an occupation outside the home has little to do with Islam.

Hazrat Ammara Naseebah, an Ansari, had the gift of healing and was known to take surgical decisions at a time when medical science had not yet developed and training was unavailable (Razwy 2014). The people of her tribe were at a loss on how they should label a woman like her, and whether they should entirely trust her diagnoses. On meeting her after his migration from Mecca to Medina, Prophet Muhammad (PBUH) acknowledged her skills and elevated her to the status of first Surgeon-General of Islam (Haykal 1976). She had been given permission to follow the army in Uhud to serve the wounded but she ended up fighting in the battle and saving the lives of many men, including that of the Prophet's when there was a shortage of soldiers. She was not just an honoured surgeon and a warrior, but also a wife and a mother. Hazrat Ammara Naseebah is a good example of how Islam permits the management and balancing of multiplicity of roles and relations for women. As the findings in my book will reveal, many women practitioners in Pakistan today are prevented from participation in governance so that they can give priority to their family and household.

Shifa bint Abdullah was a famous medical practitioner from the Quraish tribe, who at birth was named Layla (Ansari

& Nadvi 2001). Over time, as she became famous for her expertise and knowledge of preventive medicine, she began being called *shifa* or healer. Prophet Muhammad (PBUH) honoured her by asking her to teach one of his wives to read, write, and share her skills of healing with other members of society (Khan 2016). Her experience and counselling skills as a physician gave her rich expertise to deal with other social problems. The Prophet had entreated his male companions to utilize her services for the administration of public health and education services in the developing Muslim community. The fact that Shifa bint Abdullah was married with children and yet was able to successfully undertake her physician's role with success in the Prophet's time is yet another example of how married women with particular skills were promoted to assume leading administrative positions.

Rufaida Aslamiah was an Ansari from Medina, who welcomed Prophet Muhammad (PBUH) when he migrated from Mecca and is popularly known as the first Muslim nurse (Hussain 1981). Rufaida's father was a physician and with his tutelage, she became a diligent and committed healer. She is recognized for her innovation in converting her makeshift medical camp into a mobile unit which permitted her to reach the sick. In Medina, the Prophet organized a medical camp for her close to his mosque so that he could regularly visit the camp and inquire about her work. He also instructed her about aspects of Islam and healing to allow her knowledge base to expand and thereby enabling her to disseminate it to others. He also encouraged her to serve orphans and non-Muslims in the community. Not only was Rufaidah a practising nurse, but also, with the encouragement of the Prophet, a teacher who opened her own nursing school in which she trained other women to become *awasi*[9] or nurses. Rufaidah and her trainees followed the Prophet with his permission and blessings into many defensive battles for Islam. For her services, she and the other nurses were paid the same remuneration as that of male soldiers. The lesson that the Prophet left behind for his followers was that a woman nurse was an integral community worker and that she deserved equal social standing and compensation as male workers.

Umm-e-Aiman bint Tha'labah was the foster mother of Prophet Muhammad (PBUH) and she played an active role in the defensive battles of Islam by helping to nurse the wounded and providing healing services to the ailing (Ghadanfar 2001). She took active part in the battle of Khyber in view of the shortage of male soldiers. Given her experience, she was known to head the logistical planning in management and care-provision of the disabled and diseased, both in times of war and peace. Rabee' bint Mauwth was another Muslim woman who broke traditional stereotypes by being included in the Prophet Muhammad's (PBUH) close advisory circle (Ghadanfar 2001). She not only performed nursing tasks on the battlefield but also travelled back and forth between Medina and the battle sites to deliver dead bodies to their families at the Prophet's command. It is clear from the historical records of Rabee' bint Mauwth that in contrast to what is projected by conservative theology, working women in Islam are permitted to travel long distances alone unaccompanied by male relatives as guardians. They may also handle dead bodies and carry heavy physical burdens if inclined and physically fit to do so.

As regards the complete seclusion of women, Prophet Muhammad (PBUH), within the limits of hijab,[10] permitted many women to play important roles in the social structures of his Islamic community without their segregation from men.

The importance of women and the gender equality afforded by Islam is symbolized by the first Muslim convert, Hazrat Khadija, the wife of Prophet Muhammad (PBUH). Hazrat Khadija was the Prophet's employer prior to marriage and his trusted companion after their marriage (Gilani 2012). She donated all her resources for the cause of Islam and for the impoverished of her community. No record suggests that her participation in work and interaction with men was not permitted by Islam. Hazrat Fatima is known to have 'fought courageously' like a 'little tigress' to defend her father[11] and also to have spoken in a public address to the first caliph of Islam in the presence of an assembly of men, demanding the return of her usurped property (Ghadanfar 2001). There were several other Muslim women who were known to have instructed male members of society in Islamic jurisprudence and laws, and spoken in public assemblies, such as Fatima bint Khattab, Umm-e-Salim, Umm-e-Hakim, Umm-e-Shareek Dosiah, and Umm-e-Saad bint Saad. It would not be incorrect to say that the strengthening of Islam's foundation by Prophet Muhammad (PBUH) would not have been possible had interaction and coordination not existed between men and women (who were not related by blood).

Rather than the sage principles of Muhammad (PBUH), Muslim women and religious minorities living in Muslim-dominated nations like Pakistan have inherited the negative approach of the Quraysh, who introduced gender violence as a fundamental part of religion and society. The intention of the latter was to establish male supremacy and maintain women as instruments of pleasure rather than of socio-economic development as Islam proposed. The historical narrations of Islam have been remembered through the exploits of the non-Muslim women rather than the Muslim companions of the Prophet. Quraysh women were known to follow their men into battle to sing and dance, insult the Muslim soldiers, and cheer on their own soldiers with sexual promises (Bodley 1970). No Islamic sect has yet come forward to empower women in terms of work participation or narrate accounts from the Prophet's time relating to the status of women healthcare practitioners. This indirectly legitimizes violence against working women in present-day Islamic societies.

Chapter 1 will traverse the literature, setting out extant empirical evidence about the status of workplace violence faced by women healthcare providers across the world and particularly in Pakistan. The cultural features of public sector hospitals in Pakistan will be reviewed in order to understand how organizational characteristics link with safety, role-fulfilment, and error-reporting of women practitioners. As many of the women practitioners in Pakistan work in the field for the lady healthcare programme, the safety of women workers in community spaces has also been examined. To supplement the limited local academic scholarship, a brief media content analysis is presented to shed light on the reality of violence faced by women practitioners. The current shortcomings of the legal system and constitutional laws in Pakistan which bolster workplace violence form the concluding section.

Chapter 2 deals with theories relating to workplace violence in the context of gender and Pakistani culture. Three broad areas will be covered to understand the causes of violence in the context of perpetrator, structure, and victim. There is a strong relationship between the role fulfilment of women practitioners and reporting of violence in the health sector. The importance of developing and sustaining a culture of reporting violence will be expanded to include theories relating to the culture of error sharing and team building, which helps to secure job satisfaction for the woman practitioner in addition to ensuring patient safety and holistic public health.

Chapters 3 presents the quantitative, and chapters 4 to 6 the qualitative findings in relation to workplace violence faced by women healthcare providers in Pakistan that I have collected over a period of five years. Systems such as SPSS and NVIVO have been used to analyse the quantitative and qualitative data sets respectively. The reliability and ethical dimensions of the research process have been strictly adhered to in terms of anonymity, confidentiality, the safety of the participants, and informed consent (Diener & Crandall, 1978). All the participants and respondents were provided the names and free services for counselling in the event of psychological disturbance in having to relive and discuss experiences of workplace violence. The coding and categorization for qualitative analysis was undertaken both through software and manually by the author and the women research assistants,to ensure the trustworthiness of data and to re-confirm the findings (Graneheim & Lundman 2004). Regular meetings were held with senior researchers for approval of the research process and to corroborate findings (Shenton 2004), while the final categorization was communicated to senior and experienced practitioners for confirmation of content validity.

The internationally standardized WHO survey has been used to collect data from 401 women practitioners across all designations and departments. Sampling was done from a total of 19 public hospitals and basic health units across two Pakistan provinces. Nationwide data could not be collected given security and permission problems, and travel and logistical uncertainties for women researchers. To fill an

important gap in an attempt to understand the reasons for
the existence and continuation of workplace violence, 59
women practitioner participants were interviewed by me
and my trained research assistants through a semi-structured
interview process. Key themes from these interviews have
been related in order to help to enhance our awareness
about the diverse and complex socio-structural causes of
workplace violence from an insider victim perspective.
The arguments are presented thematically to ensure the
anonymity of the contributors.

Chapter 5 elaborates on the liabilities of victims which
contribute to their being subject to increased risk of cyclical
violence. Social forces that encourage women to acquire a
medical degree but then prohibit them from practising the
profession are explored. Women are socialized through overt
and covert social laws to believe that they must passively
accept violence and protect the perpetrators. Finally, as victims
of violence, women practitioners have collectively developed
defence strategies of partial care delivery and veiling in order
to minimize the prospect of violence. However, in this process,
their job satisfaction, perceptions of competence, and team
building are severely compromised.

Chapter 6 examines the perceptions of male co-workers and
health administrators in relation to the causes of workplace
violence against women practitioners. The question of
administrative legacies and legal shortfalls contributing to
the sustenance of violence are addressed. However, the most
interesting part of this chapter is the clear division of men as
friends of perpetrators and members of a patriarchal network,
which indicates perhaps the reason for the continuance of
violence against women healthcare practitioners. In the eyes
of male colleagues, women are second-class professionals

against whom violence is justified. Although the organizational structure and male attitudes which promote violence are not advocated by all the men, and strong undercurrents of guilt have been evident, there is insufficient acceptance of this to mobilize male support for women's protection.

Chapter 7, the concluding unit of this book, focuses on unmapped but vital rights that women practitioners need in order to deliver services as legitimate and valuable Pakistani healthcare professionals. Improvements in policy at the constitutional, organizational, and community levels are discussed, with attention to the role of the community, media, and religious authorities as important catalysts in the improvement of socio-cultural teachings and responses to workplace violence against women practitioners.

## References

Agarwal, Gunjan, and Kapil, (2016): 'The Mistress of Spices: A Study in the Light of South Asian Traditional Therapeutic Practices', *European Journal of English Language and Literature Studies*, 4 (6), 36–52.

Akbari, Ather H, Wimal, Rankaduwa, and Adiqa K. Kiani, (2009): 'Demand for public health care in Pakistan', *Pakistan Development Review*, 141–53.

American Psychiatric Nurses Association Position Statement (2008): 'Workplace Violence', <http://www.apna.org/files/public/apna_workplace_violence_position_paper.pdf>

Ansari, Saeed, Abdussalam Nadvi, and Syed Suleman Nadvi (2001): *Women Companions of the Holy Prophet and Their Sacred Lives*, Bombay, India, Bilal Books.

Bodley, Ronald Victor Courtenay (1970): *The Messenger: The Life of Muhammad* (Greenwood Press Rpt).

Burton, Antoinette (1996): 'Contesting the zenana: The mission to make lady doctors for India, 1874–1885', *Journal of British Studies,* 35 (03): 368–97.

Chaudhury, Ranjit Roy, and Uton Muchtar Rafei (2001): 'Traditional Medicine in Asia', World Health Organization, Regional office for South-East Asia, New Delhi, SEARO Regional Publications (39).

Chew, Dolores (2002): 'The Search for Kathleen McNally and Other Chimerical Women: Colonial and Post-Colonial Gender Representations of Eurasians', *Translating Desire: The Politics and Gender of Culture in India* (New Delhi: Katha, 2–29).

Cohen, I. Bernard (1984): 'Florence Nightingale', *Scientific American,* 250 (3): 128–37.

Crowther, A. (2001): 'Why women should be nurses and not doctors—some nineteenth century reflections', University of Glasgow, Nursing and Midwifery School Seminar, Glasgow.

Dall, Caroline Wells Healey (1888): *The Life of Dr. Anandabai Joshee: A Kinswoman of the Pundita Ramabai,* (Boston: Roberts Brothers).

Dhammika, Shravasti (1993): 'The Edicts of King Asoka', Buddhist Publication Society.

Di Martino, Vittorio (2002): 'Workplace violence in the health sector', *Country Case Studies Brazil, Bulgaria, Lebanon, Portugal, South Africa, Thailand, and an additional Australian study,* Report prepared for The International Labour Office (ILO), the International Council of Nurses (ICN), the World Health Organization (WHO) and Public Services International (PSI), Geneva.

Diener, Edward, and Rick Crandall (1978): *Ethics in social and behavioral research* (Chicago: University of Chicago Press).

Ehrenreich, Barbara (2010): *Witches, midwives, and nurses: A history of women healers*, (City University of New York, New York: Feminist Press).

Forbes, Geraldine (1994): 'Medical careers and healthcare for Indian women: patterns of control', *Women's History Review*, 3 (4): 515–30.

Friedlander, Peter (2009): 'Buddhism and Politics', (Chapter 2, *Routledge Handbook of Religion and Politics*, Edited by Jeffrey Haynes, New York: Routledge).

Ghadanfar, Mahmood Ahmad (2001): *Great Women of Islam*, (Riyadh, Saudi Arabia: Darussalam Publishers).

Gilani, Sadi (2012): 'Hazrat Khadijah', *Defence Journal*, 16 (4/5): 48.

Glubb, John Bagot (1963): *The Great Arab Conquests* (London, United Kingdom: Hodder & Stoughton).

Graneheim, Ulla H., and Berit Lundman (2004): 'Qualitative content analysis in nursing research: concepts, procedures and measures to achieve trustworthiness', *Nurse Education Today*, 24 (2): 105–12.

Hassan, Syeda Mahnaz, and Fatima Farooq (2015): 'Gendered perspective of informal sector of the economy in Pakistan', *Pakistan Journal of Commerce and Social Sciences, 9 (1)*: 185–201.

Haykal, Muhammad Husayn (1976): *The Life of Muhammad* (North American Islamic Trust, American Trust Publications).

Hussain, S (1981): 'Rufaida Al-Asalmia', *Islamic Medicine*, 1 (2): 261–2.

Kashani-Sabet, Firoozeh (2005): 'Who Is Fatima? Gender, Culture, and Representation in Islam', *Journal of Middle East Women's Studies*, 1 (2): 1–24.

Kelen, Betty (1977): *Muhammad: The Messenger of God* (New York, Pocket Books).

Kelly, Jacinta, Fealy, M. Gerard, and Roger Watson (2012): 'The Image of You: Constructing nursing identities in YouTube', *Journal of Advanced Nursing*, 68 (8): 1804–13.

Khan, Sara (2016): 'Retrieving the Equilibrium and Restoring Justice: Using Islam's Egalitarian Teachings to Reclaim Women's Rights', Chapter 5 from book Sensible Religion (United Kingdome: Routledge).

Klainberg, Marilyn (2010): 'An Historical Overview of Nursing', Chapter 2 from the book *Today's Nursing Leader: Managing, Succeeding, Excelling,* (Unites States: Jones and Bartlett Learning).

Kosambi, Meera (1996): 'Anandibai Joshee: Retrieving a Fragmented Feminist Image', *Economic and Political Weekly*, 3189–97.

Margoliouth, David Samuel (1939): *Mohammed* (London: Blackie & Son Ltd.).

McNamara, Sharon A. (2010): 'Workplace violence and its effects on patient safety', *AORN Journal,* 92 (6): 677–82.

Mebrouk, Jette (2008): 'Perception of nursing care: Views of Saudi Arabian female nurses', *Contemporary Nurse,* 28 (1–2): 149–61.

Murlidhar, Paliwal, and P.S. Byadgi (2011): 'Charaka: The Great Legendary and Visionary of Ayurveda', *International Journal of Research in Ayurveda and Pharmacy,* 2 (4): 1011–1015.

Nair, Sreelekha, and Madelaine Healey (2006): 'A profession on the margins: status issues in Indian nursing', Joint Presentation by Sreelekha Nair and Madelaine Healey at the Centre for Women's Development Studies, New Delhi. Retrieved as at 20.11.16 http://archive.nyu.edu/bitstream/2451/34246/2/profession_on_the_margins.pdf

Ohnuma, Reiko (2006): 'Debt to the mother: a neglected aspect of the founding of the Buddhist nuns' order', *Journal of the American Academy of Religion,* 74 (4): 861–901.

Ordoni, Abu Muhammad (2014), *Fatima the Gracious* (Qum, Iran: Ansariyan Publications).

OXFAM 'Ending Violence against Women': Retrieved as at 20.11.16 https://www.oxfam.org/sites/www.oxfam.org/files/ending-violence-against-women-oxfam-guide-nov2012.pdf>

Razwy, Sayyid Ali Ashgar (2014): *A Restatement of the History of Islam and Muslims* (Lulu Press, Inc).

Sehrawat, Samiksha (2013): 'Feminising Empire: The Association of Medical Women in India and the Campaign to Found a Women's Medical Service', *Social Scientist*, 41 (5/6): 65–81.

Seneviratna, Anuradha (1995): *King Aśoka and Buddhism: Historical and Literary Studies* (Buddhist Publication Society).

Shariati, Ali (2014): *Fatima is Fatima* (Lulu Press, Inc).

Shenton, Andrew K (2004): 'Strategies for ensuring trustworthiness in qualitative research projects', *Education for Information*, 22 (2): 63–75.

Smith, Cecil Woodham (1951): *Florence Nightingale* (New York City: McGraw-Hill Book Company).

Solotaroff, Jennifer L., and Rohini Prabha Pande (2014): *Violence against women and girls: Lessons from South Asia*, Washington, World Bank Group.

Spencer, Jenny S. (1989): 'Marsha Norman's She-tragedies', *Making a Spectacle: Feminist Essays on Contemporary Women's Theatre, ed. Lynda Hart* (Ann Arbor: Michigan UP), pp. 147–65.

Valiathan, M.S. (2003): *The Legacy of Caraka* (Telangana, India: Orient Blackswan).

Wilkinson, Alice (1958): *A Brief History of Nursing in India and Pakistan* (Delhi: Trained Nurses' Association of India).

Wiskow, Christiane (2003): 'Guidelines on workplace violence in the health sector', ILO WHO ICN PSI Joint Programme on Workplace Violence in the Health Sector, Geneva.

Witz, Anne (2001), 'Colonising Women': female medical practice in colonial India 1880–1890', *Clio medica*, Amsterdam: 61, 23–52.

World Economic Forum 'The Global Gender Gap Report', <http://www3.weforum.org/docs/GGGR2015/cover.pdf>

World Health Organization (2001): 'Legal Status of Traditional

Medicine and Complementary/Alternative Medicine: A Worldwide Review', Report Edited by Diane Whitney, New York.

## NOTES

1. Ayurveda originated in the fifth century BCE and is based on the theory of Panchmahabhutas. It has been widely practised in South Asia, especially in Pakistan, Bangladesh, India, Nepal, and Sri Lanka. Ayurvedic medicine includes herbal medicines and has been used to both prevent and cure diseases.

2. Unani medicine is based on the theories of Hippocrates (462–377 BCE), Galen (129–216 CE), and Avicenna (980–1037 CE). It has been widely used as the traditional system of medicine in Pakistan, China, Egypt, India, Iraq, Persia, and the Syrian Arab Republic. Like Ayurvedic medicine, Unani medicine also includes herbal medicines and has been used to both prevent and cure diseases.

3. King Asoka was the third monarch of the Mauryan dynasty. He was the first ruler of a unified India in the third century CE. After he embraced the teachings of the Buddha, he transformed his polity from one of military conquest to that of Dharmavijaya (victory by righteousness and truth). He was popularly known for the socio-political improvements he instituted and the protection he afforded to the elderly, children, women, and the sick.

4. Though the Charaka texts have contributed significantly to medical science, it is unclear whether Charaka was a man or a community. Famous physicians prior to the second century CE were usually referred to as Charaka.

5. The Dufferin Fund was set up nationwide across colonial India to construct hospitals for women patients, pay expenses for poor women patients, and provide scholarships for women studying medicine.

6. Zenana hospitals were intended only for women to enable their seclusion in order not to compromise the segregation norms of society. They were largely used to provide maternal health and gynecological services.

7. Women companions such as Aslamiah Umem Mattaa, Umm-e-Kabshah, Hamnah bint Jahash, Muaaathah, Ammaimah, Umm-e-Ziad, Rabia bint e Muawath, and Umm-e-Atiyah.

8. Women companions such as Umm-e-Atiyah, Asma bint Abu Bakr, Umm-e-Sad Kabshah.

9. *Awasi* is the Arabic word for nurse.

10. Hijab means the covering of a woman's hair, chest, and overall figure so as not to display her physical attributes to men who are not her close blood relatives. In many cases, hijab is used in front of most male blood relatives (such as uncles and cousins), apart from the husband and father.

11. From physically abusive perpetrators such as Abu Jahl bin Hisham, Shaibah bin Rabee'ah, Oqbah bin Mu'eet, and Omayyah bin Khalaf.

# 1

# The Women Healthcare Profession
# in a Patriarchal World

This chapter reviews local and international scholarship to assess the reality of workplace violence against women healthcare practitioners. There are only three health journals[1] published from Pakistan, as cited in the report by Thomson Reuters on internationally approved and accredited journals, and virtually all of the articles in these concern medical studies or case reports and not violence or organizational culture. There are no journals that address the development and problems relating to women nurses, lady healthcare workers (LHWs), and women doctors in Pakistan. Notwithstanding this dearth of literature, there was sufficient material available in international journals emphasizing that violence is a persistent problem for women in Pakistan. Some of the material used for this chapter was published by journals that are not ranked in the Thomson Reuters's report. This does not mean that the data is incorrect but that the material published has not been authenticated by a peer review.

Let us begin by defining workplace violence as briefly and broadly as possible. The debate between scholars regarding conceptual definitions of violence will not be joined in order to maintain a simple and inclusive theoretical framework.

# Definitions and Types of Workplace Violence

Gender violence in the workplace is any act that results in physical, sexual, verbal, or psychological harm to women, including threats of such acts, coercion, or arbitrary deprivation of liberty (Cruz & Klinger 2011). The salient point here is the inclusion of the word 'gender', rather than 'women', an indication that movement has been made to include in definitions the understanding that gender is a social construct that varies from region to region. The social expectations and positions of women in Pakistani society are influenced by patriarchal ideologies, and thus the phenomenon of violence needs to be examined from a gender perspective.

There are three broad types of workplace violence: verbal, physical, and sexual. For the data collection for this book the conceptual definition of violence by the World Health Organization has been used (Chappell & Di Martino 2006). Laws in the developed world still do not concur on the description and explanation of workplace violence; the consensus is that broader definitions are better because they leave room for additions and improvement (O'Leary-Kelly et al. 1996). Women healthcare practitioners face the most violence in the hospital setting, principally from three types of male perpetrators: co-workers, patients, and family attendants.

Verbal violence includes verbal harassment, humiliation, exclusion, social undermining, bullying, incivility, and a lack of respect for the dignity of an individual. No matter what the specific type, the overall construct of verbal violence remains the same. It is the least reported and least acknowledged type of violence. In most cases it is considered insignificant as covert occupational socialization is an essential part of the hidden curriculum. It is important to recognize that the hidden curriculum inculcated by medical and nursing students during training and by practitioners on the job is instrumental in the condoning and acceptance of violence against women healthcare practitioners. Young practitioners receive occupational socialization specific to the region and culture to which they belong.

However, international research suggests that consistent bullying, marked exclusion, and random one-off verbal jibes against women healthcare practitioners have significant negative consequences (Einarsen & Mikkelsen 2003; Hutchinson et al. 2006; Jackson et al. 2002; Yamada 2008). Not only are victims made to feel that they are unimportant members of the team, but they also feel disempowered to provide optimal care services. Perpetrators of verbal violence aim to generate fear and an ethos of hostility amongst women healthcare practitioners, and therefore the provision of care and emotional support becomes difficult, if not impossible. Verbal violence against women healthcare practitioners is not just an interpersonal conflict or a random act occurring infrequently; rather, it is a consistent and systematic frame of oppression imposed by perpetrators to bully and keep women in their place in order to establish a male control hierarchy.

Physical violence includes both mild and severe forms of physical assault including pushing, pinching, biting, slapping, kicking, stabbing, shooting, and homicide. Fear of physical injury is obviously a barrier to the role output and life functions of women healthcare practitioners, not merely at the workplace but also when they return home (Bennett & Robinson 2000; Bowling & Beehr 2006). A minor physical assault can leave the victim in a state of shock and deprive them of power and control in a work environment where, by definition, they need to be in control to save lives. Severe physical violence against women can cause adverse outcomes for their health, including mental anxiety and permanent physical damage. The latter can include chronic body pain, frequent headaches, impaired functioning of limbs or speech, loss of hearing or vision, a miscarriage, or other permanent disabilities. Some research even shows that women healthcare practitioners, even when working in a health centre, seek the least medical attention for physical harm they have received for fear of reporting, embarrassment, and also lack of time (Jackson et al. 2002). Exposure to workplace violence also keeps women healthcare practitioners in a constant state of anxiety of facing danger and entrapment because, as specialized professionals, they cannot easily leave a job or apply for a transfer.

Sexual violence includes unwanted, unreciprocated, and unwelcome behaviour of a sexual nature that is offensive (Anderson 2002; Fitzgerald 1993). It includes attempted or completed forced penetration or rape. Sexual advances and sexist comments about women healthcare practitioners are considered the norm in medical schools and clinical work areas. As discussing or reporting sexual violence is taboo in regions like Pakistan, victims usually resort to extended absenteeism and even leave the job or the profession altogether. Low reporting is also due to the difficulty in differentiating between blurred lines of sexual harassment and attempted aggressive courtship, and also the difficulty of defining sexual violence. Thus, whereas rape is considered sexual violence, sexual harassment is not perceived as a violent act by most people in Pakistan (Niaz 2003).

# Workplace Violence: A Global Predicament

International literature tells us that one in every three women faces some form of violence in their lifetime (OXFAM 2012). The most vulnerable targets of violence are not just women within the homes but women working in male-dominated work environments. Women care providers working in the health sector have been identified as facing high rates of violence in comparison to their male counterparts (Di Martino 2002). Some scholars estimate that healthcare providers are 16 times more at risk of facing workplace violence in comparison to other professionals (Elliott 1997). Gender violence is caused by socio-cultural classifications and imbalances of power. Women across the world enjoy lower status, opportunities, and power, which relegate them to subservient roles at the workplace and helps legitimize violence against them. There are no standardized indicators for measuring workplace violence across countries, and reports vary, with some countries having no official records of violence faced by women healthcare providers (Mayhew & Chappell 2007). Workplace violence has the effect of reducing role delivery, job satisfaction, and care-provision in healthcare practitioners across the world (Cooper & Swanson 2002).

According to official reports, workplace violence in the health sectors of developed countries such as the UK (National Audit Office 2003), US (Behnam, et al. 2011; Fasanya & Dada 2016), Canada (K. L. Hesketh et al. 2003), and Australia (Mayhew & Chappell 2003) is commonplace, frequent, and acutely problematic. Research from the West indicates too that healthcare providers working in the psychiatry (Bowers, et al. 2009) and emergency (Behnam et al. 2011) departments as young trainees (Hahn et al. 2012) and as community workers (Hanson et al. 2015) face regular and frequent incidents of violence. A systematic review of the literature confirms that workplace violence against healthcare providers is directed more towards nurses than doctors (Taylor & Rew 2011). In many developed countries such as Canada and Australia, healthcare workers have left their jobs to avoid the regular incidence of violence at the workplace and also because they have little faith in the accountability systems (Hegney et al. 2006; K. L. Hesketh et al. 2003). It has also been reported that care providers are reluctant to report violence due to fears of penalization and job loss (Mayhew & Chappell 2001).

Developing countries have, as expected, high rates of workplace violence in the health sector (Di Martino 2002). Again, records for the rate and frequency of violence are scarce, given rare and inconsistent measurement methods. Diverse scholarship suggests that China (T. Hesketh et al. 2012; Pai & Lee 2011), Taiwan (Chen et al., 2008), Iran (Teymourzadeh et al. 2014), Palestine (Kitaneh & Hamdan 2012), and other developing countries (Martino, 2002) have a high prevalence of workplace violence against women healthcare workers. Countries with regressive cultures against women and patriarchal domination have even higher incidents of workplace violence (Shoghi et al. 2008). Male-domination in health care administration and clinical structures has the effect of sustaining existing legal and governance failures, causing distress to victims and clients seeking care provision (DeSouza & Solberg 2003). Studies suggest that reporting workplace violence, and especially sexual violence, in developing countries with conservative and patriarchal cultures is very low, as victims do not want to compromise their family honour (Merkin & Shah, 2014). The consequences for women practitioner victims of workplace violence vary in terms of psychological and physical health (Gerberich et al. 2004), job satisfaction, and commitment (Boyle & Wallis 2016), and community and family involvement.

The sub-facet of healthcare services which the world is most concerned about is the level of patient safety culture (Cooper 2000). Research indicates that the practise of safety culture and the level of error commission[2] in the hospital setting can influence healthcare costs and optimal care delivery of practitioners (Mayo & Duncan 2004). Hospital organizations with an ideal patient safety culture have open co-worker communications, strong teamwork, autonomous decision-making, resource adequacy, and a tendency to blame the system rather than the individual (Pronovost et al. 2003). One of the principal constructs of this book is that violence faced by women practitioners is not merely an individual or organizational problem but also a public health concern. When women healthcare practitioners face greater violence, they: (a) commit more errors at the workplace, and (b) do not report errors made by themselves or their co-workers given fears of retribution. Lack of informal and voluntary error-sharing between co-workers, subordinate employees, and different medical specialists has negative consequences on patient safety, health recovery, and mortality.

In the developed world, hospital organizations have formal error-reporting and tracking systems, with accountability bodies to prevent adverse events. Magnet hospitals[3] aggressively train and educate healthcare professionals about the 'human element' in error-making and encourage a no-blame culture to encourage error-reporting (Lok & Crawford 1999). This notwithstanding, the high level of error-reporting in the developed world is a cause of concern, and experts suggest that even with error-tracking systems in place, it is the culture of reporting and the security and comfort of healthcare providers at the workplace which guarantees higher error-reporting and patient safety. Of concern is that the developing world lags behind in terms of the absence of laws for the protection of women healthcare practitioners and error-tracking systems.

Women practitioners globally, and in developing countries such as Pakistan, are more easily accused of committing errors, given their negative identity, low professional status, lack of resource allocation for educational advancement, and the absence of care plans (Almutary & Lewis 2012; Bayazidi et al. 2012; Donchin et al. 1995; Gorini et al. 2012; Handler et al. 2007; Lawton et al. 2012; Park 1 et al. 2011; Throckmorton & Etchegaray 2007; Unver et al. 2012; Uribe et al. 2002). The predicament for women practitioners in countries like Pakistan is further exacerbated by socio-cultural barriers against working women, such as low social status, violence at the workplace, an absence of structural support, an inefficient healthcare sector, and the absence of a system or culture of error-reporting (Khowaja et al. 2008; Rabbani et al. 2009). The introduction of anonymous reporting systems in culturally-led societies such as Pakistan has been recommended (Bayazidi et al. 2012). Anonymous reporting eliminates the possibility of retribution and also secures patient safety. However, even if challenges of reporting errors are overcome through anonymous channels, one of the root problems causing errors in the hospital will remain unchallenged unless violence against women practitioners is mitigated. This is because the high rate of workplace violence against women practitioners in Pakistan negatively influences their practise of patient safety. Women practitioner victims end up committing more errors in the hospital organization, resulting in misdiagnosis, prolonged illness, expense, and even mortality (Chapman & Styles 2006).

## Workplace Violence: The Existing Scholarship from Pakistan

Pakistan is one of the most populated countries in the world, with the tenth largest labour force. Comprising half the population, at approximately 90 million, women have the potential to become a strong human resource base for Pakistan's development. Unfortunately, grave shortages of women healthcare practitioners are prevalent there. There are several barriers which prevent recruitment and retention of women practitioners in the health sector, such as substandard work environments, inadequate pay, lower hiring quotas by government, the inferior social status of the nursing profession, and high rates of violence (Islam 2002; Kline 2003). Unlike the general impression, the Taliban are not restricted to the Afghan border, Khyber Pakhtunkhwa Province (KPK), and Karachi. They exist in small pockets across Pakistan and exert influence across most cities (Abbas 2014). The social barriers that the Taliban have franchised against Pakistani women include: (a) preventing them from attending schools, (b) restricting them from participating in the workforce, and (c) thwarting their rights to opt for child vaccination (Din et al. 2012). Many structures, including the public sector in the urban areas, under the influence of Talibanization, support the removal of women from educational and work opportunities, claiming that this enhances their security and survival. Consequently, working women, especially care providers, who interact with non-relative males face a severe backlash in the form of violence from a fundamentally regressive culture that has been given a new life by the Taliban and other such extremist groups.

Apart from the negative influence of the Taliban, there are other strongly regressive politico-cultural forces operating within Pakistan which contribute to the oppression of women workers. According to Ali and Gavino (2008), both Pakistani urban and rural communities are powerfully influenced by tribal and feudal culture. This culture strongly promotes violence against women and specifically against working women to continually remind them not to forget their place of subservience and subordination in a male-dominated social order. The commonest and popularly repeated belief system passed on from one male generation to another is that the source of all evil is *zan, zar, zameen* or woman, money, and land (Roy 1984). Not only does this ideology inculcate in men the belief that women are the repositories of all evil but it also legitimizes any force and aggression used by men against women within the homes, workplaces, and public areas. Many tribal leaders have used Islam to reaffirm their belief in condoning violence against women, and also employed shaming tactics against men who do not as a community norm openly practise aggression against women.

With such macro-cultural forces at play, it is of interest to understand, from an agency perspective, what individual Pakistani men feel about violence against women. In a study by Fikree and his colleagues (2005), married men were interviewed from diverse socio-economic backgrounds in order to find out their attitudes to wife beating and physical abuse of women. Men from the vegetable market, private hospitals, and top management executives from private clinics were interviewed, covering respondents from low to high income groups and illiterate to highly literate categories. Of the 176 male respondents, over half of them admitted to being: (a) victims of corporal punishment as children, and (b) witnesses to violence against their mothers. Nearly half of them agreed that husbands had the religious right to discipline and physically beat their wives. Given their illiteracy, it may not be surprising that men from the lower income bracket felt this way, but it is disturbing that 46 per cent of the sampled male medical practitioners believed that wife beating was acceptable. The results from this study have some important implications; first, that male practitioners may also feel that abusing women colleagues is acceptable, and second, that many more men may covertly support violence against women but not feel comfortable reporting their beliefs during interviews.

Pakistan's LHWs belong to the lower strata of society and they reside and work in underprivileged areas, outside the confines of a formal organization and at community doorsteps (A. Khan 2008). This means that LHWs are highly vulnerable targets as solitary women workers in patriarchal communities that have no standards of security. They face extreme stigmatization for providing what is considered by conservatives to be Western medical services that are violative of traditional and religious social health patterns (A. Khan 2011). The belief that the reproductive and health decisions of women and children are a private family matter has given an inferior and outsider status to LHWs. They, together with their families, face regular shaming for being employed in a profession which provides assistance in birth control and abortions. Many have been murdered and face extreme violence in the course of their daily work (Shirkat Gah and UN 2007). Mediums like the radio and religious sermons are commonly used by community notables to condemn LHWs and incite male public to abuse them (Din et al. 2012). LHWs have in some cases been unable to continue with their work due to a religious fatwa passed by the Taliban stating that it was a man's duty to kidnap LHWs and then to either kill her, marry her forcibly, or use her as a sex-slave. Besides, as the homes, dispensaries, and routes for the functioning of LHWs are public knowledge, perpetrators have found it easy to subject them to frequent violence.

Unlike the LHWs, women nurses in Pakistan largely work within clinical settings. However, because nurses also suffer from an inferior socio-professional identity, they are not immune to common and frequent victimization. Somani and Khowaja (2012) conclude in a report that the high prevalence of workplace violence against nurses exists due to feminization of the profession and a general lack of respect for women in the society. It was documented that nurses were frequently the targets of rape, sexual harassment, physical violence, and bullying at the hands of patients, family attendants, paramedical staff, and co-workers. There is a grave problem of under-reporting and lack of formal policy mobilization for the protection of women healthcare practitioners, given fears of social stigma, further violence, and job loss. Another study by Somani and colleagues (2015) confirmed that nurses suffered from bullying and mobbing behaviour at the hands of their supervisors. Indeed, horizontal bullying by senior women colleagues and women supervisors can contribute to the ineffective mobilization of women practitioner safety. In the same study, the construct of sexual harassment was also measured. Nurses indicated that they suffered from sexual harassment at the hands of male family attendants and co-workers. Other studies from Pakistan confirm that sexual violence is a norm against women practitioners (N. Khan et al. 2015b).

Lee and Saeed have also studied the oppression and violence faced by women nurses in Pakistan (Lee & Saeed 2001). They describe how the legacy of colonization has led to sustained and historical patterns of marginalization of minority groups such as women from the lower socio-economic strata. This would include nurses, LHWs, and lady doctors from rural districts and disadvantaged families. Organizational marginalization can lead to weak control and power for women practitioners in terms of work autonomy and role delivery. Issues of wage exploitation were also discussed, with the implication that lower paid women employees held lower socio-professional status, justifying violence against them. Other researchers from the region have confirmed the extreme levels of violence faced by female nurses and women health practitioners across Pakistan (Meghani & Sajwani 2013). The lack of a congenial work environment and low remuneration has forced qualified nurses to immigrate, contributing to the brain drain and nurse shortage in Pakistan (Khowaja 2009).

In a study by A.J. Khan, Karmaliani, and Ali (2015), both female nurses and doctors were sampled in order to assess how much violence they faced in a tertiary-care hospital. The respondents indicated that 97 per cent of them suffered from verbal abuse and 60 per cent suffered physical violence. The principal response of the victim practitioners was to remain silent for fear of inviting even greater violence. In another study by Mirza and colleagues (2012), a survey was conducted across nine tertiary-care hospitals in Pakistan to assess the rates of violence and abuse experienced by doctors during care delivery. From a total of 675 doctor respondents, nearly

80 per cent confirmed that they had faced some form of violence in the previous two months.

Another study by Imran and colleagues (2013) attempted to investigate aggression and violence experienced by doctors and nurses in a public sector hospital. 74 per cent of the respondents confirmed that they suffered from aggression and violence during the past 12 months. Verbal and physical violence were listed as the commonest forms of victimization, with family attendants cited as the most common perpetrators. The emergency department was cited as the most high-risk zone for practitioners and some of the reasons for the perpetration of violence were listed as resource shortages, overcrowding, and incompetent care provision. Interestingly, it was also indicated that violence was precipitated by negative media stereotypes against public sector health services, which prompted patients and attendants to resort to violence even when there was little reason to do so. It has been shown that certain specialists, such as psychiatrists, also face high rates of harassment and bullying in the region (Gadit & Mugford 2008). Most practitioners do not however take any action against the perpetrators because they feel that abuse is in the nature of their profession and thus should be accepted as a given.

Violence faced by doctors and nurses in four large tertiary-care hospitals of Pakistan was investigated by Zafar and colleagues (2013). Their findings revealed that 73 per cent of health practitioners had experienced verbal violence and 17 per cent had been subject to physical violence over the past 12 months. The following groups of practitioners were less likely to report that they had faced violence: (a) doctors in comparison to nurses, and (b) practitioners who had been working for a longer number of years. This may be so because both have more to lose in terms of socio-professional status and suffering public ignominy after reporting violence. Qureshi and her fellow scholars (2012) have theorized that nurses and other junior women practitioners are given lower status and respect in society because they are away from their homes at night and interact with unrelated males (Qureshi et al. 2012). While interviewing nurses from Sindh, it was found that sexual violence was commonly faced by women at the workplace and that none of them were aware of which organization to approach for redressal or who to seek help from when confronted with sexual assault. Junior doctors, patients, and attendants were listed as principal perpetrators and it was mentioned in the qualitative findings that violence against women practitioners was an acceptable norm in Pakistani society.

The adoption of coercive and bureaucratic styles of management by the top male executives can provide invisible and visible support for violence against women employees. Healthcare policies and investment has only benefited male practitioners and management as opposed to women healthcare practitioners, especially nurses and LHWs. Jhatial and colleagues (2013) have researched top management working in the public sector of Pakistan and found that they play a central role in practising and condoning workplace bullying and violence in order to sustain their hierarchical order, especially against subordinates and women. Senior managers were found to believe that their coercive and bullying leadership styles against women were a norm of Pakistani organizational culture because they felt a more flexible and gender-neutral approach would reduce their clout and effectiveness. Other researchers recommend that the quality of care by women practitioners could be greatly enhanced

through participatory decision-making and teamwork and
through praise and support by the leadership (Ghaffar et al.
2000).

Male healthcare providers, paramedical staff, and
administrators are known not just to practice neglect, but also
to physically and sexually abuse women patients who are not
looked after by family attendants. This is due to an absence of
monitoring and penalization in the healthcare sector and also
strong cultural currents of permissibility of violence against
women. Though incidents of sexual violence against women
patients and practitioners in the hospital setting are common,
there is almost no reporting of such aberrations. Women
victims are reluctant to disclose victimization given the grave
repercussions of inviting family dishonour and social stigma
(K. Ahmad 1999). The Pakistani male-dominated culture has
a history of incarcerating victims of rape, domestic abuse,
and workplace harassment with punishments ranging from
extreme castigations like public flogging, honour killing, and
stoning, to milder chastisement such as denial of the crime,
divorce, and ostracization or dismissal from their occupation
(Shaheed & Hussain 2007). Jetha and Punjani (2014) found
that women healthcare practitioners rarely report sexual
violence when subjected to it during clinical investigations.

Naveed et al. (2010) add that women victims of violence
suffer from guilt and that they have over time contributed
to the violence directed at them. The underlying ethos and
overt instruction by the seniors and instructors deter female
practitioners from ever reporting harassment, bullying, or
violence at the workplace. In this context, there is a serious
problem of an internalization of deservability by the latter.
Women do feel humiliated and shamed for suffering violence
silently, but feel that they will suffer much greater long-

term and permanent shame if they publicly disclose their victimization. Other studies highlight that women doctors and nurses suffer immense mental and psychological strain due to workplace violence and an inability to alter their circumstances or seek retribution (Sadia & Farooqi 2011).

## Media Reports

The Pakistani media intermittently reports one-off stories about regular beatings, homicide, and rape faced by women healthcare practitioners. A brief content analysis from newspaper articles published over the past five years reveals innumerable cases of rape, homicide, sexual harassment, and physical assault against women doctors, nurses, and LHWs. The women healthcare practitioners whose cases have received one-time news coverage after facing violence have not, however, had the satisfaction of follow-up coverage or of the perpetrators having been sentenced. In many instances, such practitioners reported suffering sexual harassment and rape at the hands of administrative heads to which they were meant to report violence and seek justice. The following cases are especially noteworthy because the inquiry committees exonerated the male perpetrators in view of their high positions and connections: (1) in June 2013, a woman doctor lodged a complaint about being gang-raped by her chief medical officer and his four accomplices,[4] (2) in July 2010, a woman nurse from Jinnah Hospital, Karachi, was raped and made to jump off the first storey of a doctors' mess by the male medico-legal officer,[5] and (3) in June 2014, a woman nurse from Hayatabad Medical Complex was sexually harassed by the deputy medical superintendent, but her appeal was dismissed by the Director General Health.[6]

Not only were instances of male co-workers getting away with assault against women practitioners common,[7] but the recurring betrayal of the Hippocratic Oath and the exploitation of vulnerable women patients by male practitioners was also confirmed by news reports.[8] Media estimates suggest that as many as 38 per cent of women doctors have left the profession nationwide over the past few years due to societal pressures and family disapproval of their practising an unsafe profession.[9] Notwithstanding insistence that the medical profession has a high status and women doctors enjoy a comparatively better standing than other women healthcare practitioners (such as nurses and LHWs), reports of regular beatings were common, not just by co-workers, patients, and family attendants[10], but also by political and state representatives.[11] Social media hacking and cybercrime had also been used as a tool of harassment against 200 women doctors.[12] Incidents of rape and violence against nurses were rampant.[13] There was also coverage of the ruthless beating of 100 unarmed women nurses by the police.[14] The assault had the purpose of stopping the nurses from protesting against the unfair dismissal of a woman colleague. Media coverage of this incident was approved by the government to communicate a harsh warning to women practitioners about the state response to protests. Most alarming was the media representation of the violence faced by LHWs, with perpetrators including police officials and regional armed forces.[15] Incidents of victimization against LHWs, such as rape and aggression against family members, were widespread[16] and in many cases the acts of violence were used in order to force LHWs to leave the profession.

# Legal Status for Working Women

Nearly half of Pakistan's population comprises women (NIPS 2013). Notwithstanding this, the legal structures and the constitution of Pakistan are dominated by feudal, tribal, and traditional laws which are weighted against justice for women. Historically, laws in Pakistan such as the Hudood Ordinance of 1979 and the Qanoon-e-Shahadat Ordinance 1984,[17] the FATAs Frontier Crimes Regulations of 1901,[18] and the Nizam-e-Adl in KPK[19] of 2009, have combined to create a fear psychosis amongst women by: (a) inculcating a sense of guilt for having experienced violence, and (b) the belief that they will never be able to prove their innocence in a punitive society (R. Imran 2013). As there is scarcely any reporting of violence against women in Pakistan, its widespread occurrence is shrouded in mist. Also, in the cases of violence which are reported, very few perpetrators are caught and punished. In 2015, Pakistan was ranked second-last from among 145 countries on the gender gap index, highlighting that our women suffer critical inequalities in accessing health and education, economic opportunities, and political representation.

In 2015, the Senate of Pakistan passed a resolution on Working Women's Day to provide safe and secure, harassment-free workplaces for women. Prior to this, the Harassment of Women at the Workplace Act was passed in 2010. It is not that political resolve has not been shown but that Pakistani women do not have any awareness and social support to use the existing laws to punish and deter perpetrators. Balochistan and KPK still do not abide by the Act and have not appointed ombudspersons to deal with complaints of harassment. Sindh has ombudspersons but the reportage of violence is minimal.

This is due to discriminatory clauses and exclusions in the law which continue to handicap the case for women's protection. The act is criticized for its inefficacy in: (a) not providing *suo motu* power to the local ombudsman to help women who have little knowledge of the law, (b) not including in the definition of 'workplace' educational institutions, hostel areas, employer accommodation, public areas, and private homes where field workers (like LHWs, paramedical staff, and physiotherapists) provide services, and (c) not including in the definition of 'harassment' the commission of any objectionable or inappropriate act, comment, or display which causes injury, insult, or humiliation, and the creation of a hostile work environment.

In 2016, Punjab became an example for other provinces by introducing the Punjab Protection for Women against Violence Act. The Act provides civil remedies such as protection orders, residence orders, and monitory orders, and this represents the first focused state initiative to recognize and protect working women. However, the Act has several flaws which need amendment before it can become a source of protection for both working and non-working women. There are no separate clauses recognizing that working women suffer violence and that they need special protective measures. In the definition of 'perpetrators of domestic violence', there is no allowance for non-blood relatives and men to whom women victims are not married. This excludes women healthcare practitioners who face violence from co-workers, patients, and family attendants within their homes, hostels, and in hospital-provided accommodation. The protection orders of the act do not take into consideration that third party accomplices of the perpetrator can also victimize a woman in her home, place of shelter, or at the workplace.

Alarmingly, the Act includes a clause for the imprisonment and fining of women who make false accusations but it does not take into consideration that legitimate victims can be forced to accept that they have made a 'false accusation' under the duress of perpetrators. Currently, men who torture their wives are not sentenced to jail and this can become an incentive for perpetrators to re-victimize women who dare to report violence. GPS trackers have been introduced to trace previous offenders, but the tracker cannot deter perpetrators who have not been caught in the past and technological malfunctions can render the tool ineffective. The toll-free complaint number for victims and the contact numbers for the rescue teams have not been extensively advertised and most of the women in Punjab seem to be unaware of its existence. The Violence Against Women Centres (VAWC) aimed to assist victims in filing complaints against perpetrators and providing medical assistance and shelter for victims are not currently visible or accessible. Also, the specific locations and the number of VAWC across the province have not been specified. There is no mention of provisions in the VAWC for daughters and special needs children who would need shelter with the victim mothers. The Act permits Women Protection Officers (WPO) to enter any house, at any time, to rescue a victim. However, there is a risk that WPOs can be harmed during this exercise and there needs to be provision for armed male police officers to accompany the women officers on such rescue missions. Another big hurdle preventing the Act from becoming operational and effective is the religious leadership. The Council for Islamic Ideology, Jamaat-e-Islami, and Jamiat Ulema-e-Islam have all vehemently opposed the Act by terming it un-Islamic and warning that it can destroy Pakistan's family system.

There can never be justice or safety for women without the support of all the religious leaders in Pakistan. Unfortunately, notwithstanding the introduction of laws, the fear is that the police will never follow through on investigating violence against women, the judicial system will not provide justice to women complainants, and political and tribal authorities who uphold strong male networks will protect perpetrators. Signing international charters and attending global summits for gender equality like the United Nations Convention on the Elimination of All Forms of Discrimination Against Women (CEDAW) are formalities that hold little relevance and are ineffective in altering cultural norms and traditional beliefs. It is only the indigenous transformation of norms and beliefs that can alter laws and have them implemented.

To secure national and provincial legislative improvements and implementation of laws, there needs to be greater representation of women in healthcare governance, hospital administration, overall politics, and public offices. Thus far, informal and semi-formal justice mechanisms have failed to secure protection and justice for working women victims. A female doctor or nurse at the hospital must report victimization to her supervisor or the medico-legal officer, whereas an LHW will report to her Lady Health Supervisor (LHS). In the hospital an inquiry committee may be set up if the case is serious and media hype is created but in most cases the Head of Department (HoD) or supervisor will off-the-record defuse the event and advise the victim to accept violence as a norm. Victims will be castigated for bringing the incident out in the open and attempting to defame the profession and their family honour. Although justice and accountability can also be mobilized through the Young Doctors Association (YDA) and the Young Nurses Association

(YNA), the most these bodies have yet been able to achieve is temporary strikes and minor gains in terms of compensation. Pakistan's formal laws blatantly favour men. This, in all probability, is one of the principal reasons for the low female labour participation ratio in the country. Apart from regressive social norms barring women from working, male guardians remain fearful that the lack of security provided by the socio-legal structures will place the women of their families at risk when they enter the workplace. The official constitution and legal features of Pakistan support informal social laws and traditional norms which subjugate women and it is this inequality that remains a precursor to violence. A married woman cannot apply for a passport, obtain a national identity card, or register a business without her husband. Similarly, many women cannot demand equal inheritance rights. There are no women in the constitutional courts of Pakistan[20] and the quotas for women seats in local government is very low at 33 per cent (Drage 2001), given that the female population ratio is nearly equal to men.

Most working women in Pakistan carry the social burden of singlehandedly taking care of children, parents, in-laws, and sick relatives (Bari 2000, A. Khan 2007). There is no state law providing child allowance for parents or entitlement to leave to care for sick relatives. Some of the workplace laws, as outlined by the Women, Business, and Law Report, 2016, keep women in subordinate positions and highlight how they are structurally discriminated by depriving them of: (1) equal pay, (2) gender neutral hiring, (3) prohibition on enquiries about family status, (4) equivalent positions and promotion after maternity leave, (5) entitlement to breaks and spaces for lactating mothers, and (6) part-time work hours for homemakers and mothers with dependent children. There are over 70 laws in Pakistan dealing with employers' rights (I. Ahmad 2009), however, none deal directly with violence against women healthcare practitioners, and this is a significant reason for low reporting by women victims and prosecution of perpetrators. Alarmingly, the Punjab and Sindh Ministry of Law and Justice have no reported cases of harassment against women between the years 2012 and 2015 (Human Rights Commission of Pakistan 2016). LHWs and nurses have been unable to tackle the issue of violence and safety because of critical deficit in salaries and service structure. Not getting paid for months at a time or earning low incomes has forced women practitioners to focus all their efforts on strikes for equitable compensation. In most cases they have had to return to work due to pressures from administration and government, with the minor benefit of getting paid their arrears or gaining trifling increments. The law that protects women from being dismissed for taking a maternity break does not have provisions for securing her position and promotion when she returns to work and consequently many women with several children have to suffer displacement and a lack of advancement. Although Article 37(e) of the Labour Rights Provision claims that the state will secure just and humane working conditions for women and the 2010 Protection of Women against Harassment Act requires public and private organizations to adopt an internal code of conduct and establish a complaint cell, there has been a complete lack of follow-up and accountability in relation to both of these measures. It is obvious that without central and provincial government surveillance and penalization, an internal code of conduct for complaints and appeal will not become operational and effective within individual hospitals.

Mobilization by women leaders for legal reform in Pakistan's recent history has not been a success. Indeed, such women have become victims themselves. Numerous women rights' activists, in their pursuit of improvements, have endured state sanction, threats to themselves and members of their families, sexual violence, and discrimination at the hands of political, military, and religious leaders. Widely circulated news of women rights activists becoming targets of violence have served as disincentives and warnings to other women attempting to pursue similar initiatives for the protection of women. This includes prominent community notables, non-government organization (NGO) activists, media personnel, lawyers, journalists, and political representatives, such as: (1) Farida Afridi, co-founder and human resource manager of Society for Appraisal and Women Empowerment in Rural Areas and a Pashtun feminist, was murdered in 2012 by the Taliban, (2) Asma Jehangir, who helped to form the Women's Action Forum and is a former chairperson of the Human Rights Commission of Pakistan, was beaten in 2005 by state police for attempting to raise awareness of issues concerning violence against women, (3) Samar Minallah Khan, a social documentary film-maker and the founder of an independent media think tank called Ethnomedia, was forced to go into hiding after facing multiple death threats from the Taliban,[21] (4) Khawar Mumtaz, (the CEO of a women's rights NGO called Shirkat Gah), Sarah Zaman (the Director of the NGO named War Against Rape), and Tabassum Adnan (the founder of the women-only *jirga* named Khwendo Jirga), along with their workers receive threats and regularly face physical abuse, (5) Marvi Sirmed, a journalist and human rights activist, was threatened with rape and physical harm by a prominent member of the Jamiat Ulema-e-Islam party on live television,[22] and (6) Dr Arfa Syeda Zehra, Chair of the National Commission on the Status of Women, Government of Pakistan, and a member of the Law and Justice Commission of Pakistan, received multiple threats against continuance of her work in support of women's rights.

## Conclusion

A combination of academic literature review and media content analysis confirms that there is systematic and frequent violence against women practitioners globally and in Pakistan in particular. Shortages of women in the health sector and the overall labour force of Pakistan can be overcome by enhancing the protection and status of women providers. Ease of access and financial concessions makes public sector hospitals the primary service provider for a majority of the poor and illiterate people in Pakistan. However, extremely low government budget allocations have compromised on the quality of services provided by the public sector, causing dissatisfied users to become explosively violent against women practitioners, as women will always remain easier targets in non-punitive environments. Feminized professions like nursing and the lady healthcare programme specifically suffer the most violence and also high impact physical and sexual abuse. LHWs deliver services to impoverished and illiterate communities where they have to interact with unregulated and conservative men. In public spaces where women are expected to remain within the home and in purdah, the LHWs are viewed as radical agents who are delivering services which compromise the traditional control over health and reproduction.

Male physicians and administration wield overwhelming power in controlling workplace decisions, including standards of respect and security for women workers. Male patriarchal supremacy in the organization has led to diverse organizational problems for women practitioners, including inadequate staffing and resources, inadequate training by medical lecturers and clinical instructors, limited autonomy and control, lack of higher education and career advancement, lack of benefits and provisions for working mothers, absence of communication and teamwork between different practitioners, and nonexistent care plans and error-reporting systems. A range of academic reports suggest that over 70 per cent of women practitioners in Pakistan are subject to violence of one form or another, with up to 97 per cent encountering verbal abuse, and up to 60 per cent suffering from physical violence. The most salient finding was the lack of reporting of violence by women practitioners and the belief of nearly half of a group of sampled male practitioners that beating women is acceptable.

To compound the problem, women from the lower classes face even greater inequality and violence at the workplace, are given inferior social classifications, and are unable to mobilize support for justice. Women will always remain an easier target in Pakistan given the regressive cultural norms which legitimize violence against the weaker gender. Structural failures coupled with an inherently patriarchal organizational culture in Pakistan have resulted in inequality and subjugation for its working women. Media reports confirm that violence is rampant and also that, more alarmingly, male perpetrators are almost invariably exonerated given strong patriarchal networks. Male practitioners not only imposed violence on women co-workers but also on vulnerable women patients. Male perpetrators include high ranking male medico-legal officers, chief medical officers, medical superintendents, the Director

General of Health, political representatives, and police officers, making it virtually impossible for women to resist and report violence or bring the culprits to book. From a public health standpoint, there is concern that when women practitioners experience violence, it negatively influences patient mortality and safety. Workplace violence against women practitioners can cause cyclical violence because victimized women become incapable of providing optimal care delivery for the public, and consequently this can encourage additional violence against them from an aggravated public and co-workers.

## References

Abbas, Hassan (2014): *The Taliban Revival: Violence and Extremism on the Pakistan-Afghanistan Frontier* (New Haven: Yale University Press).

Ahmad, Iftikhar (2009): 'Labour and Employment Law: A Profile on Pakistan', ILO Memo.

Ahmad, Khabir (1999): 'Public protests after rape in Pakistani hospital', *Lancet*, 354 (9179): 659–59.

Ali, Parveen Azam, and Maria Irma Bustamante Gavino (2008): 'Violence against women in Pakistan: a framework for Analysis', *Journal of the Pakistan Medical Association* 58 (4): 198.

Almutary, Hayfa H., and Peter A. Lewis (2012): 'Nurses' willingness to report medication administration errors in Saudi Arabia', *Quality Management in Healthcare,* 21 (3): 119–26.

Anderson, Cheryl (2002): 'Workplace Violence: Are some nurses more vulnerable?' *Issues in Mental Health Nursing,* 23 (4): 351–66.

Bari, Farzana (2000), 'Women in Pakistan: Country briefing paper', Asian Development Bank.

Bayazidi, Snor, et al. (2012): 'Medication error-reporting rate and its barriers and facilitators among nurses', *Journal of Caring Sciences*, 1 (4), 231.

Behnam, Marcelina, et al. (2011): 'Violence in the emergency department: a national survey of emergency medicine residents and attending physicians', *Journal of Emergency Medicine*, 40 (5): 565–79.

Bennett, Rebecca J., and Sandra L. Robinson (2000): 'Development of a measure of workplace deviance', *Journal of Applied Psychology*, 85 (3): 349.

Bowers, Len, et al. (2009): 'Identifying key factors associated with aggression on acute inpatient psychiatric wards', *Issues in Mental Health Nursing*, 30 (4): 260–71.

Bowling, Nathan A., and Terry A. Beehr (2006): 'Workplace harassment from the victim's perspective: a theoretical model and meta-analysis', *Journal of Applied Psychology*, 91 (5): 998.

Boyle, Malcolm J., and Jaime Wallis (2016): 'Working towards a definition for workplace violence actions in the health sector', *Safety in Health*, 2 (1): 4.

Chapman, Rose, and Irene Styles (2006): 'An epidemic of abuse and violence: nurse on the front line', *Accident and Emergency Nursing*, 14 (4): 245–49.

Chappell, Duncan, and Vittorio Di Martino (2006): *Violence at Work* (Geneva, International Labour Organization).

Chen, Wen-Ching, et al. (2008): 'Prevalence and determinants of workplace violence of health care workers in a psychiatric hospital in Taiwan', *Journal of Occupational Health*, 50 (3): 288–93.

Cooper, C., and Naomi Swanson (2002): 'Workplace violence in the health sector', State of the Art Conference, Geneva: International Council of Nurses.

Cooper M.D. (2000): 'Towards a model of safety culture', *Safety Science*, 36 (2): 111–36.

Cruz, Adrienne, and Sabine Klinger (2011): *Gender-based violence in the world of work: Overview and selected annotated bibliography*, Working Paper, Bureau for Gender Equality, Geneva: International Labour Office.

DeSouza, Eros R., and Joseph Solberg (2003), 'Incidence and dimensions of sexual harassment across cultures', *Academic and Workplace Sexual Harassment: A handbook of cultural, social science, management, and legal perspectives*, pp. 3–30, United States of America, Praeger Publishers.

Di Martino, Vittorio (2002): 'Workplace violence in the health sector', *Country Case Studies Brazil, Bulgaria, Lebanon, Portugal, South Africa, Thailand, and an additional Australian study*. Report prepared for The International Labour Office (ILO), the International Council of Nurses (ICN), the World Health Organization (WHO) and Public Services International (PSI), Geneva.

Din, Iftikhar Ud, Zubia Mumtaz, and Anushka Ataullahjan (2012): 'How the Taliban undermined community healthcare in Swat, Pakistan', *BMJ*, 344, e2093.

Donchin, Yoel, et al. (1995): 'A look into the nature and causes of human errors in the intensive care unit', *Critical Care Medicine*, 23 (2): 294–300.

Drage, Jean (2001): 'Women in Local Government in Asia and the Pacific—A comparative analysis of thirteen countries', Report for United Nations Economic and Social Commission for Asia and the Pacific.

Einarsen, Stale, and Eva Gemzoe Mikkelsen (2003): 'Individual effects of exposure to bullying at work', *Bullying and emotional abuse in the workplace: International perspectives in research and practice:* 6.

Elliott, Pamela P. (1997): 'Violence in Healthcare', *Nursing Management*, 28 (12): 38–42.

Fasanya, Bankole K., and Emmanuel A. Dada (2016): 'Workplace violence and safety issues in long-term medical care facilities: Nurses' perspectives', *Safety and Health at Work*, 7 (2): 97–101.

Fikree, Fariyal F., Junaid A, Razzak, and Jill Durocher (2005): 'Attitudes of Pakistani men to domestic violence: A study from Karachi, Pakistan', *The Journal of Men's Health & Gender*, 2 (1): 49–58.

Fitzgerald, Louise F. (1993): 'Sexual harassment: Violence against women in the workplace', *American Psychologist*, 48 (10): 1070.

Gadit, A.A.M. and G. Mugford (2008): 'A pilot study of bullying and harassment among medical professionals in Pakistan, focusing on psychiatry: need for a medical ombudsman', *Journal of Medical Ethics*, 34 (6): 463–66.

Gerberich, Susan Goodwin, et al. (2004): 'An epidemiological study of the magnitude and consequences of work-related violence: the Minnesota Nurses' Study', *Occupational and Environmental Medicine*, 61 (6): 495–503.

Ghaffar, Abdul, Birjees Mazher Kazi, and Mohammad Salman (2000): 'Health care systems in transition III. Pakistan, part I. An overview of the health care system in Pakistan', *Journal of Public Health Medicine*, 22 (1): 38–42.

Gorini, Alessandra, Massimo Miglioretti, and Gabriella Pravettoni (2012): 'A new perspective on blame culture: An experimental study', *Journal of Evaluation in Clinical Practice*, 18 (3): 671–75.

Hahn, Sabine, et al. (2012): 'Patient and visitor violence in the general hospital, occurrence, staff interventions and consequences: a cross-sectional survey', *Journal of Advanced Nursing*, 68 (12): 2685–99.

Handler, Steven M., et al. (2007): 'Identifying modifiable barriers to medication error-reporting in the nursing home setting', *Journal of the American Medical Directors Association*, 8 (9): 568–74.

Hanson, Ginger C., et al. (2015): 'Workplace violence against homecare workers and its relationship with workers health outcomes: a cross-sectional study', *BMC Public Health*, 15 (1): 11.

Hegney, Desley, et al. (2006), 'Workplace violence in Queensland, Australia: The results of a comparative study', *International Journal of Nursing Practice*, 12 (4): 220–31.

Hesketh, Kathryn L, et al. (2003), 'Workplace violence in Alberta and British Columbia hospitals', *Health Policy*, 63 (3): 311–21.

Hesketh, Therese, et al. (2012): 'Violence against doctors in China', *BMJ*, 345 (sep07 1), e5730–e30.

Human Rights Commission of Pakistan 'Women: Rights of the Disadvantaged', <http://hrcp-web.org/hrcpweb/wp-content/uploads/2016/04/Women_12.pdf>

Hutchinson, Marie, et al. (2006): 'Workplace bullying in nursing: towards a more critical organisational perspective', *Nursing Inquiry*, 13 (2): 118–26.

Imran, Nazish, et al. (2013): 'Aggression and violence towards medical doctors and nurses in a public health care facility in Lahore, Pakistan: A preliminary investigation', *Khyber Medical University Journal*, 5 (4): 179–84.

Imran, Rahat (2013): 'Legal Injustices: The Zina Hudood ordinance of Pakistan and its implications for women', *Journal of International Women's Studies*, 7 (2): 78–100.

Islam, A. (2002) 'Health sector reform in Pakistan: Future Directions', *Journal* of the *Pakistan Medical Association*, 52 (4): 174–82.

Jackson, Debra, J. Clare, and J. Mannix (2002): 'Who would want to be a nurse? Violence in the workplace—a factor in recruitment and retention', *Journal of Nursing Management*, 10 (1): 13–20.

Jetha, Zohra Asif, and Neelam Saleem Punjani (2014): 'Rape: Crime Hidden under Social Stigma', *International Journal of Science and Research*, 3 (6).

Jhatial, Ashique Ali, et al. (2013): 'Psychopathy in Management

Behaviour and Bullying at Work: Hearing some unheard voices from Pakistan', *Gomal University Journal of Research*, 29 (1).

Khan, Ayesha (2007): 'Women and paid work in Pakistan', *Pathways of Women's Empowerment* (Karachi: Collective for Social Science Research).

Khan, Ayesha (2008): 'Women's empowerment and the lady health worker programme in Pakistan', *Karachi: Collective for Social Science Research*.

Khan, Ayesha 2011: 'Lady Health Workers and Social Change in Pakistan', *Economic and Political Weekly*, 46 (30): 28–31.

Khan, Azmat Jehan, Rozina Karmaliani, and Tazeen Saeed Ali (2015a): 'Interpersonal Verbal and Physical Abuse against Female Nurses and Doctors in Karachi, Pakistan', *International Journal of Nursing Education*, 7 (2): 290–5.

Khan, Noor, Begum, Shabina, and Shaheen, Ashrat (2015): 'Sexual harassment against staff and student nurses in tertiary-care hospitals Peshawar KP Pakistan', *International Journal of Innovative Research and Development, ISSN* 2278–0211, 4 (1).

Khowaja, Khurshid (2009): 'Healthcare systems and care delivery in Pakistan', *Journal of Nursing Administration*, 39 (6), 263–5.

Khowaja, Khurshid, et al. (2008): 'A systematic approach of tracking and reporting medication errors at a tertiary-care university hospital, Karachi, Pakistan', *Therapeutics and Clinical Risk Management*, 4 (4): 673.

Kitaneh, Mohamad, and Motasem Hamdan (2012): 'Workplace violence against physicians and nurses in Palestinian public hospitals: a cross-sectional study', *BMC Health Services Research*, 12 (1): 469.

Kline, Donna S (2003): 'Push and pull factors in international nurse migration', *Journal of Nursing Scholarship*, 35 (2): 107–11.

Lawton, Rebecca, et al. (2012): 'Identifying the latent failures underpinning medication administration errors: An exploratory study', *Health Services Research*, 47 (4): 1437–59.

Lee, Marilyn B., and Ismat Saeed (2001): 'Oppression and horizontal violence: The case of nurses in Pakistan', *Nursing Forum* (36: Wiley Online Library): 15–24.

Lok, Peter, and John Crawford (1999): 'The relationship between commitment and organizational culture, subculture, leadership style and job satisfaction in organizational change and development', *Leadership & Organization Development Journal*, 20 (7): 365–74.

Martino, Vittorio di (2002): 'Workplace violence in the health sector: Country case studies of Brazil, Bulgaria, Lebanon, Portugal, South Africa, Thailand, and an additional Australian study'.

Mayhew, Claire, and Duncan Chappell, (2001): *Occupational violence: Types, reporting patterns, and variations between health sectors* 139, (NSW: School of Industrial Relations, University of New South Wales).

Mayhew, Claire, and Duncan Chappell (2003): 'Workplace violence in the health sector: A case study in Australia', *Safety*, 19: 6.

Mayhew, Claire, and Duncan Chappell (2007): 'Workplace violence: An overview of patterns of risk and the emotional/ stress consequences on targets', *International Journal of Law and Psychiatry*, 30 (4): 327–39.

Mayo, Ann M., and Denise Duncan (2004): 'Nurse perceptions of medication errors: what we need to know for patient safety', *Journal of Nursing Care Quality*, 19 (3): 209–17.

Meghani, Shaista Rajani, and Salma Sajwani (2013): 'Nursing: a profession in need in Pakistan', *I-Manager's Journal on Nursing*, 3 (3): 1.

Merkin, Rebecca S., and Muhammad Kamal Shah (2014): 'The impact of sexual harassment on job satisfaction, turnover intentions, and absenteeism: findings from Pakistan compared to the United States', *Springer Plus*, 3 (1): 215.

Mirza, Nabil Mahmood, et al. (2012): 'Violence and abuse faced by junior physicians in the emergency department from patients and their caretakers: a nationwide study from Pakistan', *Journal of Emergency Medicine*, 42 (6): 727–33.

Naveed, Anila, Ambreen Tharani, and Nasreen Alwani (2010): 'Sexual harassment at workplace: are you safe?', *Journal of Ayub Medical College*, 22 (3): 222.

Niaz, Unaiza (2003): 'Violence against women in South Asian countries', *Archives of Women's Mental Health*, 6 (3): 173–84.

NIPS, II (2013): 'Pakistan Demographic and Health Survey 2012–13', Islamabad.

O'Leary-Kelly, Anne M., Ricky W, Griffin, and David J. Glew (1996): 'Organization-motivated aggression: A research framework', *Academy of Management review*, 21 (1): 225–53.

National Audit Office, Great Britain (2003): *A Safer Place to Work: protecting NHS hospital and ambulance staff from violence and aggression*. Report by the Controller and Auditor General, Prepared for the House of Commons, London, The Stationary Office.

OXFAM, 'Ending Violence against Women', <Retrieved as at 20.11.16 https://www.oxfam.org/sites/www.oxfam.org/files/ending-violence-against-women-oxfam-guide-nov2012.pdf>

Pai, Hsiang-Chu and Sheuan Lee (2011): 'Risk factors for workplace violence in clinical registered nurses in Taiwan', *Journal of Clinical Nursing*, 20 (9–10): 1405–12.

Park, et al. (2011): 'Survey of Factors Associated with Nurses' Perception of Patient Safety', *Asian Pacific Journal of Cancer Prevention*, 12: 2129–32.

Pronovost, P.J., et al. (2003): 'Evaluation of the culture of safety:

survey of clinicians and managers in an academic medical center', *Quality and Safety in Health Care,* 12 (6): 405–10.

Qureshi, Misbah Bibi, et al. (2012): 'Coping with Sexual Harassment: the Experiences of Junior Female Student Nurses and Senior Female Nursing Managers in Sindh Pakistan', *The Women: Annual Research Journal of Gender Studies*: 4.

Rabbani, Fauziah, et al. (2009): 'Culture and quality care perceptions in a Pakistani hospital', *International Journal of Healthcare Quality Assurance,* 22 (5): 498–513.

Roy, Shibani (1984): 'Concept of Zar, Zan and Zamin: A Cultural Analysis of Indian Islamic Tradition of Inheritance and Kinship', *Man in India Ranchi,* 64 (4): 388–96.

Sadia, M., and Nilofer Y. Farooqi (2011): 'Workplace harassment and post-traumatic stress symptoms among Pakistani female doctors and nurses', *Inter-disciplinary Journal of Contemporary Research In Business,* 3 (6): 56–69.

Shaheed, Farida, and Neelam Hussain, (2007): *Interrogating the Norms: Women Challenging Violence in an Adversarial State* (Colombo, Sri Lanka, International Centre for Ethnic Studies).

Shirkat Gah and United Nations (2007): 'Talibanisation & Poor Governance: Undermining CEDAW in Pakistan: Second Shadow Report', Lahore: Shirkat Gah. Retrieved as at 20.11.16 http://shirkatgah.org/shirkat/wp-content/uploads/2017/01/Talibanization-and-Poor-Governance-English.pdf.

Shoghi, Mahnaz, et al. (2008): 'Workplace violence and abuse against nurses in hospitals in Iran', *Asian Nursing Research,* 2 (3): 184–93.

Somani, Rozina, et al. (2015): 'Sexual Harassment towards Nurses in Pakistan: Are we Safe?', *International Journal of Nursing Education,* 7 (2): 286–89.

Somani, Rozina and Khurshid Khowaja (2012): 'Workplace violence towards nurses: A reality from the Pakistani context', *Journal of Nursing Education and Practice*, 2 (3): 148.

Taylor, Jessica L., and Lynn Rew (2011): 'A systematic review of the literature: workplace violence in the emergency department', *Journal of Clinical Nursing*, 20 (7–8): 1072–85.

Teymourzadeh, Ehsan, et al. (2014): 'Nurses exposure to workplace violence in a large teaching hospital in Iran', International Journal of Health Policy Management, 3 (6): 301–5.

Throckmorton, Terry, and Jason Etchegaray (2007): 'Factors affecting incident reporting by registered nurses: the relationship of perceptions of the environment for reporting errors, knowledge of the nursing practice act, and demographics on intent to report errors', *Journal of PeriAnesthesia Nursing*, 22 (6): 400–12.

Unver, Vesile, Sevinc Tastan, and Nalan Akbayrak (2012): 'Medication errors: perspectives of newly graduated and experienced nurses', *International Journal of Nursing Practice*, 18 (4): 317–24.

Uribe, Claudia L., et al. (2002), 'Perceived barriers to medical-error-reporting: an exploratory investigation', *Journal of Healthcare Management*, 47 (4): 263.

Yamada, David C. (2008): 'Workplace bullying and ethical leadership', *Journal of Values-Based Leadership*, 1 (2): 49.

Zafar, Waleed, et al. (2013): 'Healthcare personnel and workplace violence in the emergency departments of a volatile metropolis: results from Karachi, Pakistan', *Journal of Emergency Medicine*, 45 (5): 761–72.

## NOTES

1. Journal of the College of Physicians and Surgeons Pakistan, Pakistan, Journal of Medical Sciences, and Journal of the Pakistan Medical Association.

2.  Medical practitioner errors include: (1) a lack of attentiveness (e.g. not checking wounds and/or dressing after surgery), (2) Lack of fiduciary concern (e.g. knowledge that doctor is misdiagnosing and failure to question this to prevent patient harm), (3) Inappropriate judgement (e.g. lack of skill or knowledge or incorrect application), (4) Medication error (e.g. administration of the wrong drug or of the wrong dosage of the drug to the patient), (5) Lack of intervention on the patient's behalf (e.g. failure to provide for the patient's needs, for example advice on the mother's nutritional requirements post delivery), (6) Lack of prevention (e.g. failure to prevent harm to the patient, for example in terms of hygiene and infection), (7) Mistaken senior doctor's orders (e.g. missing or mistaking a work order and thereby causing harm to the patient), and finally, (8) Documentation errors (e.g. error in making an entry in the chart or failure to make a relevant entry altogether. There are four error-induced possibilities described by literature: (1) error prevented from reaching patient, (2) error did not cause harm, (3) error caused some harm, and (4) error caused adverse event.

3.  A term developed by the American Nursing Council, a magnet hospital has characteristics of high patient safety and low patient mortality. The reasons for this have been found to include higher quality of care, greater nursing autonomy, and an optimal organizational culture (with greater teamwork, training, and safety for practitioners and patient).

4.  *Pakistan Gender News,* 12 July 2013; website: http://www. pakistangendernews.org/rape-accused-being-cushioned-by-pia-probers/

5.  *The Express Tribune,* 16 July 2010; website: http://tribune.com.pk/ story/28187/medical-report-says-jpmc-nurse-was-raped-dna-test-results-awaited/

6.  *The News International,* 2 August 2015; website: https://www.thenews. com.pk/print/54242-hmc-nurse-accuses-dms-of-sexual-harassment

7.  a. *Pakistan Gender News,* 30 August 2015; website: http://www. pakistangendernews.org/tag/workplace-harassment/
    b. *The Express Tribune,* 08 September 2014; website address: http:// tribune.com.pk/story/759340/nurse-shares-harrowing-tale-of-sexual-harassment/

8.  a. *The Express Tribune,* 17 October 2015; website address: http://tribune. com.pk/story/974664/on-camera-doctor-on-the-run-after-caught-sexually- molesting-female-patients/
    b. *Pakistan Today,* 11 April 2016; website: http://www.pakistantoday.

com.pk/2016/04/11/national/male-nurse-rapes-20-year-old-girl-patient-at-pimss-icu/

c. *Aaj News*, 14 May 2016, website: http://aaj.tv/2016/05/rape-allegation-on-siuts-doctors-management-refused/

9. *Samaa News*, 21 August 2015, website: http://www.samaa.tv/health/2015/08/38-lady-doctors-quit-profession-in-past-5-years/

10. *The Express Tribune*, 26 August 2011; website: http://tribune.com.pk/story/239626/medical-drama-manhandled-female-doctors-at-sobhraj-want-to-wrap-up-the-issue/

11. *Current Affairs Pakistan*, 12 July 2013; website: http://www.currentaffairspk.com/pml-n-mpa-arif-sandhela-slapped-lady-veterinary-doctor-sana-sheikhupura/

12. *Daily Times*, 4 April 2016; website: http://dailytimes.com.pk/pakistan/04-Apr-16/200-lady-doctors-blackmailed-by-using-mobile-phone-application

13. a. *Pakistan Today*, 4 February 2015; website: http://www.pakistantoday.com.pk/2015/02/04/city/lahore/body-of-raped-and-murdered-mayo-nurse-found/

b. *Pakistan Gender News*, 19 November 2014; website: http://www.pakistangendernews.org/doctor-booked-raping-nurse/

14. *Dawn News*, 17 March 2014; website: http://www.dawn.com/news/1093742

15. Asian Human Rights Commission, 5 January 2016; website address: http://www.humanrights.asia/news/urgent-appeals/AHRC-UAC-001-2016

16. *Dawn News*, 27 December 2015; website: http://www.dawn.com/news/1229421

17. The Hudood and Qanoon-e-Shahadat Ordinance (or Law of Evidence), were introduced in an attempt to bring state laws under Shariah or the injunctions of Islam, as interpreted by Sunni Hanafi doctrines. Rulings penalizing the act of rape required women victims to provide four male witnesses to prove their innocence. Many women complainants and rape victims, falsely accused of fornication and adultery, were subjected to harsh and sometimes inhuman punishments such as imprisonment, whipping, amputation, and stoning to death through the misuse of these laws.

18. The Frontier Crimes Regulations (FCR) are part of a set of special laws that govern the Federally Administered Tribal Areas of Pakistan (FATA). The FCR does not allow the Pakistani parliament's authority

to interfere in the laws and convictions passed by FATA leaders. The FCR law prohibits FATA inhabitants from rights of: (1) appealing against a conviction, (2) legal representation, and (3) presenting reasoned evidence. Women in FATA have suffered the most because the FCR laws have been grossly misused in cases where false accusations were made.

19. The Nizam-e-Adl is an order of justice approved by the Pakistan government to allow Shariah law to be practised in Malakand division, an administrative part of the Khyber Pakhtunkhwa (KPK) province. Misinterpreted laws of Islam are applied by this justice system to severely oppress women.

20. The Supreme Court of Pakistan (SCP) is the head of the judicial system in the country. It comprises a Chief Justice (selected by the President) and a number of other judges. The SCP has final authority over the Apex Constitutional Courts (one for each province: The High Courts of Lahore, Sindh, Balochistan, Peshawar, and Islamabad), and settles constitutional disputes relating to gender violence, women's protection, and workplace violence. Pakistan is the only country in South Asia to have never appointed a woman Supreme Court judge.

21. Samar Minallah Khan had released the footage of a girl in Swat being flogged by the Taliban. The girl had been flogged with the authorization of the commissioner of Malakand and thus by releasing the video, and attempting to raise international censure, Samar had become a target for both politicians and the Taliban.

22. Vile abuse was also levelled at Marvi Sirmed's mother during the live television diatribe. The perpetrator, notwithstanding graphic proof, was never held accountable, publicly denounced, or penalized for his threatening behaviour.

# 2

# Theories of Workplace Violence

Theories of workplace violence enable the researcher to understand how societies and organizations allow violence to function in specific and complex ways. The theories underlying this chapter come from the fields of sociology, public health, and gender research to provide a multidimensional theoretical perspective in order to understand why violence occurs against women health practitioners, specifically in countries like Pakistan. Women professionals are front line practitioners in the hospital setting, interacting with diverse co-workers from different specialties, and also with the wider society. Violence against women in the hospital setting and in public zones is influenced by the policies of the healthcare sector, society's views about women practitioners' identity, and community norms relating as a whole to the treatment of working women. Social norms, male attitudes, laws and policies, and misinterpretation of religious texts all contribute to making women healthcare practitioner's soft targets for violence.

Of concern is that when women practitioners face violence it has a serious negative impact on their role delivery and patient safety. In order to identify permanent solutions to the elimination of violence against women in the health sector, theories that assess why violence against women occurs at the workplace need to be explored. No particular theories can be found to explain why South Asian and Muslim women healthcare practitioners face violence but there are a number of generic theories, from which an academic discussion has been developed to explain the causes, greater risks, and likely precipitators of violence against women healthcare practitioners in Pakistan. These theories explore organizational weaknesses and the likely characteristics of perpetrators who are likely to perpetrate violence, and also the characteristics of women victims who as subjugated and passive recipients invite sustained violence.

## Perpetrator Theories

Psychological theories focus on individual acts which drive violence, and encompass both perpetrator and victim behaviour. Sigmund Freud's work presents three important arguments about man's basic nature: (a) that he is inherently anti-social and has no love for either his neighbour or enemy (Freud 1930), (b) that it is in his basic nature to use force and violence to satisfy his sexual needs (Freud 1918), and (c) that societies express their unity through conflict and the imposition of violence on common enemies (Freud 1967). On the basis of this Freudian theory we may deduce that men in general not only have a natural instinct to be violent against women but might also consider women to be their common enemy. In societies like that in Pakistan, where traditional norms regulate women within their homes, men inflict violence on working women both because it is in their nature to be violent and also because they want to protect the patriarchal social order.

John Archer argues that because sex selection is a part of

the male biological make-up, it leads to males demonstrating greater competitive and aggressive tendencies (Archer 2009). Women, especially those who resist or ignore male advances, become susceptible to greater violence. This argument is strengthened by empirical statistics which have always shown men to be more violent than women, in the homes and at the workplace, and have also shown that social conflict exists in societies with higher male ratios. Male socio-demographic characteristics which have been associated with more aggressive and violent behaviour include single status, lower economic class, and frustrated personalities. In regions like South Asia, where cultural and informal social laws take precedence over state law, violence against women can assume both biological and social prominence.

Biological theories of violence have not gained much support and this has created greater dependency on psychological, cultural, and structural explanations of workplace violence (Hesketh et al. 2003). According to Dreikur, Lew, and Bettner, misbehaviour occurs when individuals perceive their needs to be unmet by society and its organizational structures. Unmet needs may drive individuals to seek attention, gain power, and avenge themselves through violence and aggression (Lew & Bettner 2002). This argument suggests, unlike the Freudian concept of man's innate nature, that individuals are responsible for choosing their own destructive and conflict-ridden paths after their exposure to primary and secondary socialization. These choices are determined by a sense of social belonging and connection with family, parents, and early socializing agents. Family circumstances, the birth order, and siblings all contribute to the choices an individual makes between behaviour and misbehaviour. Derivatively, it may also be that patients and family attendants impose violence on women practitioners because they feel their needs have not been met in terms of care delivery and health recovery. This may be because the conditions, expertise, and resources of public healthcare facilities in Pakistan are extremely inadequate and cause the public to resort to violence against the most vulnerable targets, as women tend to be.

Carl Gustav Jung went further in order to exemplify that there is a dark side to the individual or self, which violates the ego and forces it to develop a new destructive identity (Huskinson 2002). Jung's psychological theory argues that every individual has opposing or conflicting forces within their self, and non-acceptance of the dark side of their ego may even lead to insanity. Thus, not only is violence inevitable in human nature but it is necessary to accept this darker side of the self in order to avoid complete self-destruction. It is the practice of violence which assists individuals to experience life and the development of the self. Again, culturally this may be a good theory to apply to a conflict-ridden and patriarchal state like Pakistan, where men are in a conflict between modernization and fundamentalism. Notwithstanding media and academic representation of gender equality and safety, men are strongly influenced by historical and religious traditions, and also childhood lessons from their elder male relatives, which encourage them to deal violently with women. We could also conclude that men in patriarchal communities emulate the traditional patterns of violence against women to avoid taking the risk of losing their manhood and sense of self-worth.

Social identity theory suggests that an individual defines the self in terms of group membership and how society treats and regards them (Hogg 2006). The theory highlights that the individual or professional identity of a worker would not only influence their social support system in society but also impact their structural access and empowerment. In this way, social identity has been found to influence clinical outcomes and hospital efficiency. In countries like Pakistan, women workers have a negative professional identity, especially nurses and LHWs, and this adversely influences their productivity in the hospital setting (Willetts & Clarke 2014). Nurses, LHWs, and other women healthcare workers are front line practitioners who have to deal with co-workers[1] and patients from a variety of social backgrounds. This is especially so for public sector tertiary-care hospitals in Pakistan. Public health settings are frequented by both city dwellers and rural villagers. The latter do not have access in their regions to tertiary-care hospital services provided by the state or the private sector. Therefore, women healthcare practitioners encounter patients from different social backgrounds, who are largely illiterate and strongly influenced by regressive cultural norms which consider women to constitute subordinate members of society.

Randall Collins elaborates that violence occurs through: (1) the strong and powerful upon the structurally or physically weak, and (2) by bullies upon the isolated and socially disconnected (Collins 2009). Although micro-violence may be unsuccessful over a period of time, for example, a wife who is victim to violence from her husband may leave the marriage, but with macro-violence, there may be the complexity of sustained abuse. At the organizational level, when workplace violence becomes part of the structural processes, even when the victim leaves the job, violence will still be experienced by the replacement. Public sector jobs in Pakistan are especially characterized by difficulties in entry, promotions, transfers, and complaint reporting, and this is especially for women and those lacking network connections within the higher bureaucracy. Given this, women at the workplace may both be physically and structurally disempowered to combat systematic violence against dominant male perpetrators.

The social role theory was developed to explain how gender differences influence the division of labour (Eagly et al. 2000). Women are naturally and socially expected to be caring, passive, and dependent; whereas men are expected to be controlling, aggressive, and autonomous. More specific and complex roles are developed across differing regions and communities, so whereas women in some societies may be given greater support through the symmetrical sharing of home and work roles, others remain sequestered in exclusively domesticated roles. This may result in greater social penalization and victimization for women who stray from their domesticated roles and attempt to assume autonomy in male-dominated work organizations. Eagly with Steffan further theorized that the male gender is more likely to participate in physical aggression and violence in organizations, with women as the predominant victims (Eagly & Steffen 1986). Men are expected to be tough, violent, and aggressive, and primary socialization trains them to fulfil these stereotypes through various sources such as parental training, media exposure, schooling, literature, and military conscription or athletic instruction. In organizational settings, where gender roles are allocated according to cultural expectations as they are in Pakistan, men can become more aggressive against working women, perceiving them to be violating community norms by not staying at home.

Paul Spector theorizes about counterproductive work behaviour or intentional acts which are intended to harm the employees and the fulfilment of organizational objectives (Spector 1982). Inadequate organizational conditions cause frustration and anger leading to counterproductive behaviour, such as theft, absence from work, and various forms of violence. The theory also proposes that male workers subject to external control and reporting engage in greater violence than those subject to internal control and reporting. This means that temporary employees and administrative heads reporting to external health centres may be more likely to be deviant and counterproductive. In Pakistan, there are several forces leading to extended control due to politicization, kinship networks, and the VIP culture (Islam 2004). Male practitioners and administrators with strong external networks easily get away with violence against women because they know that their privileged networks will protect them from being accountable for their misdeeds.

Edwin Megargee theorized about under-controlled and over-controlled employees and how both groups, though extremely different, can exhibit inadequate control when resorting to violence (Megargee 1966). Though it is evident how under-controlled individuals behave in rebellious and unregulated ways, the theory describes how even over-controlled people can become deviant and violent. In the hospital setting, male doctors and administrators who show qualities of meekness and conscientiousness can become aggressive and abusive. This is because rigid control and suppressed impulses over a long period of time may build up and lead to overt and explosive aggression. Dollard et al. (1939) propose that employees in an organization can become violent when they feel threatened in terms of their autonomy and professional status. The theory stresses that the stronger the threat, the greater will be the violent reaction by individuals. In addition, the force of the aggression will be more extreme when the perpetrator perceives greater satisfaction and job security post the act. In all, women practitioners can be at risk of violence from different types of male perpetrators, such as those who are highly impulsive, highly controlled, and acutely insecure in the work setting.

Mack and colleagues (1998) have discussed how stress can cause workplace violence and that stress triggers can be caused by both individual and organizational characteristics. These stress triggers can be precipitated by the inability to handle: (1) colleagues from the opposite gender, (2) patients from different cultural backgrounds, and (3) unsuitable professional choices. Individuals can also suffer great stress due to organizational problems of: (1) excessive role burden, (2) inadequate training, and (3) resource and staff shortages. Stress can cause feelings of anger, anxiety, frustration, and hostility which can lead to violent acts. Undeniably, men in countries like Pakistan may face multiple levels of stress relating to an absence of education in gender relations, political and economic uncertainty, and professional and future security fears. This may trigger tendencies of aggression and violence.

Attachment theory by John Bowlby further explains how the absence or neglect of parents in the early years can lead individuals to acts of conflict and aggression during their adult years (Bowlby 2005). The theory argues that men are less attached to and receive a lower sense of security from their mothers in comparison to their fathers who are also their principal role models for life. In Pakistan, and other patriarchal communities, men have a number of mother figures in the household, including their biological mother, aunts, grandmothers, and elder sisters, but their principal guidance and direction comes from the male heads of the household and male relatives. Because men have less attachment to women relatives, their management of relationships with women co-workers also remains unbalanced and can often manifest itself in aggressive and violent behaviour.

## Structural Theories

Workplace violence against women is reflective of the community norms of people at large and the culture of the organization. Customs and structures, specifically in regions like Pakistan, are not gender neutral and in fact violence against women workers is considered acceptable (Fitzgerald & Ormerod 1993). It is common for women healthcare practitioners to be victimized by men. Women workers in inferior organizational positions are oppressed in order to safeguard male power and control. Oppressive social structures in the home and workplace are sustained by powerful male groups who impose 'good' and 'useful' violence to maintain the social order (Toch 1993). The social investment in good violence is rewarded and preserved by patriarchal social structures because of the great pay-offs, or the patriarchal dividend, in maintaining traditions, religious authority, and cultural norms relating to a woman's role in the community.

The study of gender inequality and socially stratified professions is strongly influenced by the underlying concepts of social justice and social equality. Oppression theory suggests that individuals are stratified[2] on the basis of gender, class, religion, ethnicity, age, culture, and other variations (Kuumba 1994). Although social power remains invisible, it is a hard reality that shapes and dictates relations between two principal types of social groups: the dominant and the oppressed. Oppression against women healthcare practitioners has been empirically shown to include not just workplace bullying and professional discrimination but also violence and abuse (Hutchinson et al. 2006). There are three different levels of oppression; personal, cultural and structural, which operate as recurring forces to oppress and dehumanize women. Women healthcare practitioners are known to be oppressed at a personal level with individuals treating them as an inferior care-providers and menial workers whose task is cleaning and washing. At a cultural level, the wider community and social norms influence the relations with women healthcare practitioners in a negative manner. Cultural attitudes and practices dictate that they are treated derisively by the public, given the feminization of their profession and the assumption that women nurses, doctors, and LHWs do not provide actual medical support. Finally, at a structural level, policies and rules are created to oppress women healthcare practitioners in a systematic, cyclical, and sustained manner to deny them benefits and advancement.

Gendered role allocations include community expectations of what each gender should deliver as their professional output at the workplace (Cooper et al. 2013). As role allocations for women always entail a maternal role, women practitioners are expected to provide emotional care and passively accept any form of deviant behaviour (Anderson et al. 2001). Although there is public acceptance of women practitioners in the health sector, derived from the cultural needs of segregation, the status of women practitioners is lower than that of their male colleagues. Male healthcare practitioners are considered superior both in skill and clinical judgment, and therefore accorded greater power. Two functions come into play in Pakistan given the traditional role expectations: first, that as women healthcare practitioners are less proficient, they deserve to be discriminated against, and second, that because male healthcare practitioners have better judgement, their treatment of women colleagues is always just. The vertical and horizontal segregation of women healthcare practitioners also bears testimony to the gender inequality in the healthcare sector. There are a negligible number of women in high status administrative positions in Pakistan. Similarly, a majority of the women practitioners will be found in nursing, gynaecology, teaching of health sciences, pathology fields, or as lady health workers, and so they are under-represented in other departments of the healthcare sector. Gendered recruitment and patterns of segregation can make women healthcare practitioners more vulnerable to violence.

Albert Bandura's social learning theory describes how the observer learns and imitates the behaviour of an aggressive person, which may include parents, peers, and co-workers (Bandura 1978). Violence occurs with greater frequency in environments in which there are multiple and powerful models of aggressive behaviour. The healthcare sector is known to be a high frequency ground for violence and aggression worldwide, in comparison to any other organizational setup (Beech & Leather 2006). Individual male workers learn aggressive forms of behaviour from other men who are powerful and hold high status at the workplace. The theory also allows for the negative influences purveyed by television, video games, and other media sources which orient and depict violence and aggressive behaviour as a norm. Potential perpetrators of violence are greatly influenced by their perceptions of self-efficacy and their ability to resort to violence without fear of repercussions. The target for victimization is usually a weaker person outside the dominant power group and with a lowlier identity in society or the organization, such as women healthcare practitioners. Media reports of frequent beating, abuse, and violence being perpetrated against women healthcare practitioners in a country can encourage the practice and perpetuation of violence in the health sector.

O'Leary-Kelly, Griffin, and Grew theorize that workplace violence will flourish in a setting where it is permitted to exist (O'Leary-Kelly et al. 1996). Violence can become part of the organizational culture to such a degree that it is like a contagious disease which is passed on to anyone visiting or employed within the hospital. Normalization of violence can occur due to organizational deficiencies such as weak policies, over-crowding of patients and excessive noise, shortage of staff, inadequate resources, and unfair treatment of employees and/or patients. Aggressive and violent members of the organization, with higher status and power, can greatly influence the occurrence and sustenance of violence within the organization, and thus a combination of structural and actor violence is at play, both of which feed off each other. The status and power of violent dominant male groups in the healthcare sector of Pakistan can create spiralling imitation and reinforcement amongst other male members of the workplace, such as administration, practitioners and staff, and even patients and family attendants.

Ones and his colleagues (1993) used integrity tests to further establish the role of organizations in sponsoring counterproductive work behaviour. Constructs of integrity, such as reliability, conscientiousness, agreeableness, and emotional stability, were itemized. Those individuals found to possess greater attributes of integrity engaged in less violence at the workplace. Most of these constructs of integrity are part of an individual's personality but the theory proposes that they can be powerfully reinforced by the organization during clinical socialization. Thus, a work organization that supports partial role delivery, dishonesty, and corruption would encourage counterproductive behaviour and also violence. Researchers like Zygmunt Bauman (2010) theorize that violent work environments are compounded in their aggressive intensity because of the unwillingness of bystanders to stand up against perpetrators. Bystander inaction can contribute to the normalization of violence and cause victims to lose their confidence and feel incapable of formally reporting their victimization. The inaction of bystanders can include incidents like a senior male doctor ignoring verbal assault on nurses by patients or ward supervisors disregarding the improper advances made toward female doctors by their male subordinates.

Michel Foucault's theory of power suggests that discipline and domination in an organization occurs through legitimate and visible means (Hartsock 1990). When perpetrators of violence are not punished or held accountable, they feel that their actions are being socially and morally legitimized. In turn, victims believe their perpetrators have a right to victimize them as part of the natural social and organizational order. Foucauldian discourse suggests that the absence of violence against women would spoil the functional fit and collective harmony of an organization. Inspired by Foucault's work, Clegg (1993) proposed a circuit of power model, which describes how obedience is generated by powerful groups within an organization. Power agents are able to discipline, control, and subjugate less privileged groups. Systems within the organization operate to overcome resistance and penalize detractors for reporting violence, complaining about supervisors, and appealing for training. The bureaucratic management of the public health sector in Pakistan has been likened to an iron-cage for women practitioners who are severely handicapped in any battle for their safety and/or autonomy. Foucault and Walton's (2005) arguments highlight how cultural discourse plays a prominent role in undermining and minimizing acts of violence. Discourse and hidden curricula combine to condone violence against women. Social and organizational discourse is controlled by those in power, with discursive practice shaping knowledge and defining what is accepted across the community. Apart from labels, statuses, and role expectations, discourse also defines what violence is and what it is not.

Bies and Tripp (1996) discuss how the violation of trust in an organization can lead to revenge-led violence by perpetrators. When employees feel their trust has been violated, they begin considering themselves to be victims and therefore become aggressive in order to seek retribution for their ill treatment. Organizational conditions which can cause patients and attendants to become aggressive include inadequate care delivery, shortage of resources, and medical errors. Similarly, in the event that women practitioners report errors or a breach of conduct by male colleagues, the latter can resort to revenge-led violence. Thau, Bennet, Mitchell, and Marrs (2009) have also theorized about employees becoming deviant when they feel they have been treated unfairly or abused by their supervisors. Male healthcare practitioners, who are discriminated against by their male supervisors, may replicate patterns of abuse against vulnerable targets like their women colleagues in order to relieve their frustrations and insecurities.

As outlined by Acker (1990), the entry of women into the workplace is a cost for men, but women healthcare practitioners become necessary due to segregation and the need to provide services for female members of the community.

The organization not only recognizes men as superior employees but subjugates women employees through different means in terms of inadequate safety and remuneration. The survival and maintenance of the feudal culture in Pakistan depends upon underpaid female labour within the economy. This culture of exploitation has been transported to the workplace with women healthcare practitioners receiving comparatively inferior pay, employee benefits, and on-the-job skill enhancement. The public healthcare regime and society both benefit from women healthcare practitioners but at little cost. When women employees accept lower pay and benefits, a culture of exploitation surrounds them, in which even victimization becomes a major component. Wilson and Kelling (1982) further propose that when there is already evidence of different types of abuse and neglect in an organization functioning without accountability, it encourages individuals to participate in more acts of aggression and violence. The result is that organizations with non-punitive cultures face greater disorder when they do not develop formal and structural mechanisms to monitor, punish, and mitigate violence against vulnerable groups.

## Victim Theories

Accountability bodies and theorists have largely focused on the perpetrators of workplace violence, and ignored the aspect that victims also play a role leading to their victimization. Anne Campbell (1995) helps to assess two areas that concern this area of study: first, the reason for female acceptance of violence and second the indirect and low level of violence directed by women practitioners against female colleagues.

With the use of biological theories, Campbell concludes that because women undertake the social role of reproduction, they engage in less aggressive and more passive behaviour in order to survive and maintain their reproductive and maternal roles in life. The fear of fighting violence and losing livelihoods takes precedence as a defence mechanism to guarantee both economic and mortal survival. Campbell also proposes that women may engage in aggressive tactics like bullying not to gain status, but to secure survival (Campbell 1999). Many women healthcare practitioners in supervisory roles need to retain their jobs by participating in verbal and horizontal violence against female subordinates in order to meet the expectations of patriarchal organizational structures and to secure their positions.

Martinko and Gardner (1982) developed a model of learned helplessness to show that over time employees learn organization induced helplessness. When faced with organizational characteristics of repeated punishment, criticism, abuse, and violence, individuals, especially minority groups like women, not only underperform in their role delivery but remain helpless in the face of assault. Hence, theoretically, the expected reaction of a victim reporting incidents of violence, fighting back, and pursuing legal accountability all become alien concepts. Larwood and Wood (1977) suggest that cultural conditioning and organizational conditioning encourages passive behaviour by women and thus reduces the probability of assertive behaviour when it is appropriate. Furthermore male-dominated workplaces create hierarchies which accept derogatory language and practices against women. Overall, the norm of the organizational culture becomes to routinely tolerate bullying and harassment against women healthcare practitioners.

Stephen Schafer (1967) describes how victims have certain characteristics or elements which make them more susceptible to violence. One of these is their frequent interaction with perpetrators of violence. Women healthcare practitioners by virtue of their job are constantly in contact with their commonly evidenced perpetrators: co-workers, patients, and family attendants. Other researchers add that women who appear to be unwilling to defend and report victimization become easy targets for violence (Watson et al. 1988). Perpetrators perceive women healthcare practitioners to be powerless and fearful of losing their public honour by reporting violence, and women thus contribute to their vulnerability when facing maltreatment within the organization.

Einarsen and Skogstad (1996) suggest that the power differences between the perpetrator and victim and the victims' belief that they will be unable to gain retribution or honour after reporting the event contributes to the sustenance of violence. Communities that marginalize and defame working women also have a common culture of violence against them, and in this the victims play a prominent role. Working women accept their inferior labels and status and consider violence against them to be acceptable and common. The social, political, and cultural risk factors for violence against women are maximal in regions like Pakistan, making victims less confident of reporting and overturning patterns of systematic violence. Workplace violence is used as a weapon to relieve stress and maintain male hierarchical orders in the hospital setting. This makes it more difficult for women healthcare practitioners to defend themselves or take action to change the organizational order or policies for safety, which in turn makes them more susceptible to violence.

Leinenger and McFarland's (2002) cultural congruent

theory reasons that the ability of a woman healthcare practitioner to provide care depends upon her understanding of the cultural variations of the patient. The theory suggests that practitioner training and education must include holistic elements of not just the science of the profession but also the cultural knowledge and understanding of patient backgrounds and ethnic needs. Women healthcare practitioners who have not been trained in how to deal with patients from different socio-cultural backgrounds can face victimization. The public sector hospitals of Pakistan have an eclectic mix of co-workers and patients from different languages groups and ethnicities. In such circumstances, a lack of cultural competency training for practitioners can lead to violence and abuse against vulnerable targets like women nurses and LHWs. Also, the society is severely gender-segregated, with practitioners and the public receiving no training in how to overcome complex prejudices during interaction with the opposite gender.

Sexual harassment against women in a Muslim society will always be considered a private domain (Hussain & Khan 2008). Women healthcare practitioners have been coached by their mothers as young girls never to acknowledge or speak of commonplace sexual innuendos, sexual glances, or sexual tactility experienced by them in public. Sexual harassment against working women in a public domain is considered normal and justified, given that women are breaching a salient cultural norm by having sought employment outside the home in male territories. Not only are women viewed as sexual objects but women healthcare practitioners attired in their uniforms are commonly portrayed in pornography, cartoons, and social media as sexual objects of lust and loose morals. McKinnon (1979) suggests that within organizations sexual harassment is a significant weapon used by men to exert power. The vulnerability and fear of a woman facing sexual harassment at the workplace or in delivering services in public zones ensures that she is incapable of fulfilling her optimal role and stepping out of her bounds to achieve her maximum potential as a healthcare provider. The loss of dignity suffered after sexual harassment or violence ensures that men are able to maintain control over the output and subjugation of women co-workers.

Taylor's (1983) cognitive adaptation theory sheds light on how women victims attempt to gain control of their victimization and seek positive self-identity. A majority of women victims accept and adapt themselves to violence and then raise their self-esteem by comparing themselves to other less fortunate victims who have faced morbidity, job loss, and/or permanent physical and psychological damage. Here possibly, women also compare themselves to other women who have attempted to report or discuss violence and faced public shaming and family dishonour in the process. Thus cognitive adaptation can also become a major reason for non-reporting and sustained abuse.

## Violence and the Link to Patient Safety

One of the greatest motivators for seeking to prevent workplace violence against women globally is to produce a more supportive organizational culture in the health sector (Williams et al. 2004). Durkheim's theory emphasizes that employees of an organization must have a consensus of common goals, collective conscience, and mechanical solidarity[3] (Lincoln & Guillot 2004). In a hospital setting different specialists such as physicians, surgeons, lab-technicians, nurses, pharmacists, ambulatory care workers, and hospital administrators are highly dependent on the consensus and collaboration between one another to ensure patient safety and healthcare efficiency within the organization. Collective beliefs and attitudes within an organization determine the complex interaction between actors and the quality of production (Reeves et al. 2008). In patriarchal and misogynistic organizational cultures, women are victimized and suppressed from reporting errors, which compromises practitioner role delivery and patient safety (Estabrooks et al. 2006). The advantage that an organization has over a nation is that it can change its culture and processes more easily and over less time. In the health sector of Pakistan, improvements in organizational culture and the treatment of women workers could become harbingers of change for other structures across the country.

Rosabeth Moss Kanter's theory of power epitomizes that when workers have power in the work settings, they have the ability to get things done (Kanter Moss 1977). The theory sets out that there are informal and formal power dynamics within organizations. The formal power of a worker is officially allocated (such as governance participation) and the informal power is more culturally and socially allocated by co-workers and administrators (such as respect and dignity). Empowerment of women practitioners provides them with the ability to control role delivery, medical resources, and care structures. Research has confirmed that empowering woman practitioners in the hospital setting has positive results for their job satisfaction and patient safety (Laschinger et al. 2000). In the context of this study, it is extremely important to consider the theory of power and empowerment because a woman practitioner in Pakistan is dependent on external socio-structural forces which grant her professional autonomy.

The organizational dominance of male hierarchies can prove to be an obstacle for a woman practitioner's control over patient safety, access to adequate resources, and the freedom to report errors in the hospital setting. Foucault theorizes that nursing is a political process which combines scientific knowledge with contextualized knowledge (Gastaldo & Holmes 1999). The absorption of medical-scientific knowledge is not devoid of politics. Horizontal bullying of women healthcare practitioners results in them being sidelined in terms of education and training which means they are less knowledgeable about how to ensure optimal care delivery. The implication is that violence controls a woman practitioner's knowledge base within the organization, with serious consequences on overall patient safety. With regard to contextualized knowledge, nurses have frequent and intimate contact with patients and are informed of their family backgrounds and community problems. This combined knowledge empowers nurses to holistically treat patients. However, the degree of holistic care provided by nurses and other women practitioners is dependent on the allocators of power, including the government, health sector administrators, and hospital heads.[4] A woman healthcare practitioner habitually faced with bullying and abuse will be unable to optimally fulfil her responsibilities. She may not be able to truthfully document patient progress or provide efficient care delivery if fear of violence and her personal safety are constantly at the top of her mind.

Donabedian's (1988, 2005) structure, process, and outcome model (SPO model) is relevant in explaining the efficiency of the public healthcare sector. The model creates a prototype of quality of care to assess the performance of practitioners in a healthcare system. There are two elements in the performance of a practitioner: first, the technical skill and performance of the practitioner, and second, the interpersonal relations between the practitioner and co-workers or patients.

According to the SPO model, the measurement of the quality of care is undertaken by assessing three categories. The first is 'structure' or the work environment and resources, the second is 'process' or the care plans and procedure for practitioner and patients, and the third is 'outcome', which refers to the effect on the health of the patient. It is implied that when structures and processes are weakened by condoning violence against women employees, healthcare outcomes are plagued by inefficiency and risk to patient safety.

Agency theory describes the problems that may occur in an organization when supervisors[5] and subordinates do not cooperate with one another (Eisenhardt 1989). Sometimes the goals of the supervisor and subordinate may differ and it may be too difficult and expensive for the former to track the daily workings of the latter. Also, the risk preferences of each agent may be different which would cause them to take different actions when risk-taking in role delivery. Overall, the relationship between the principal and subordinate influences communication, promotions, job satisfaction, role delivery, and care plans. This theory directly addresses organizational efficiency at a macro-level and principal-subordinate relationship failure at a micro-level. From a gender angle, aggressive attitudes and violence by male supervisors can influence women subordinates negatively in terms of responses such as lying, blaming one another, availing of extended and repeated sick leave, leaving the job, requesting departmental changes, and non-reporting of errors. In many societies, it is the male supervisors and other authority figures who impose significant barriers against women from reporting workplace violence in order to safeguard their actions and hegemony.

Negotiated order theory helps us to better understand the maintenance of not just the social order within the organization but also the culture of error-reporting and patient safety (Strauss et al. 1963). The theory concludes that a well-negotiated relationship between male and female co-workers in the hospital setting will result in improved decision-making in terms of patient safety. Needless to say, a relationship based on conflict and violence between male and female co-workers in the health sector jeopardizes optimal role delivery on the part of the practitioners. Relevant to this study is the concept of social and organizational order which, if maintained, enables woman practitioners to perform their role optimally and consequently create an environment of error-sharing and patient safety.

Finally, Vaughn's (2004) structural secrecy theory argues that organizations embedded with layers of structural secrecy promote incomplete learning, lack of access to information, and segregated or compartmentalized knowledge. Vaughn recommends that an organization is most efficient when communication is formalized, valid, and complete. When communication within the organization is incomplete, it increases the risk of errors and dangers to patient safety. If women healthcare practitioners are victimized and not considered equal members of the care delivery team, they automatically have less access to information. In male-dominated organizations, knowledge-sharing, competency training, and strategies for professional growth become private domains for male colleagues from which women are excluded. The consequence of this is that women remain inferior and less knowledgeable team-players who can become risks for patient safety and increased error production. This can contribute to cyclical violence, hostility, and resentment against women healthcare practitioners from not just male co-workers but also dissatisfied patients.

## Conclusion

A rich theoretical framework has been developed examining the known causes and sustenance of violence against women healthcare providers. Pakistan is a conflict-ridden country with habitual violence and aggression across public spaces due to major geo-political factors. Lessons from perpetrator theories make it clear that cultural traditions, family socialization, history, and conservative interpretation of religious teachings powerfully combine to motivate men to commit violence against working women. When men have less attachment to their significant others, like immediate family members, they tend to take out their frustrations and anger on generalized minority groups such as women. Individual inability to deal with organizational conditions and high levels of stress, along with the threat of losing control can also become triggers for aggression against women at the workplace.

Notwithstanding modernization and the access to global media, religious sectarianism and eco-political instability has fuelled the polarization of gender roles and gendered spaces. Structural theories reveal that the roots of gender violence found in the public healthcare sector lie in the early primary socialization of men both within the homes and during academic training. Men learn to be aggressive and abusive towards women from elders in the family and supervisors in the clinical setting. The normalization of violence through legitimate and visible structures allows it to grow unchecked in healthcare organizations. The unwillingness of bystanders and witnesses in the health setting to stand up for victims contributes to the strengthening of structural violence and the helplessness of the victims. Organizational failures of the public sector, such as shortages of staff and resources, can encourage perpetrators to consider themselves disadvantaged and vent their frustrations through perpetrating violence against marginal groups such as women practitioners. Violence against women practitioners exists globally, but in patriarchal societies like Pakistan, it is a deliberate tool to keep working women in a position of subservience in order to maintain the traditional social order. Neo-Marxist ideologies provide incentives for feudal and élite groups in society to suppress and underpay women workers, especially those belonging to inferior classes and ethnicities of society. To prevent movements for the protection and equality of working women, they are consistently ignored and subjugated and this can be a great risk, especially in healthcare occupations which by definition require the autonomy of workers.

The concept of an 'ideal' Pakistani woman, enforced by traditions and community, is that of a passive and accepting victim. Victim theories explain that women victims are afraid that by disclosing or reporting violence they will lose their occupation and family honour. In addition, as perpetrators have greater socio-professional status and also better networks at the higher echelons of the management hierarchy, women victims have little faith in achieving retribution by reporting victimization. Frequent interaction with perpetrators in the healthcare setting and an inability to provide culture specific care for an ethnically diverse public also places the victim in more vulnerable positions.

Women in Pakistani society are unable to discuss the experiences of violence, especially of a sexual nature owing to it being a taboo subject, and therefore turn to adaptive strategies of internalizing experiences of violence. Many women practitioners even consider themselves to be fortunate in getting away with low impact and concealed violence in a region that is known for extreme and severe forms of violence. Finally, violence prevents women from performing functions expected from a professional medical practitioner and contributes to error-commission and risk to patient safety during health service delivery which further lowers the status and dignity of the woman practitioner in the workplace.

## References

Acker, Joan (1990): 'Hierarchies, jobs, bodies: A theory of gendered organizations', *Gender & Society,* 4 (2): 139–58.

Anderson, Cameron, et al. (2001): 'Who attains social status? Effects of personality and physical attractiveness in social groups', *Journal of Personality and Social Psychology,* 81 (1): 116.

Archer, John (2009): 'Does sexual selection explain human sex differences in aggression?', *Behavioral and Brain Sciences,* 32 (3–4): 249–66.

Bandura, Albert (1978): 'Social learning theory of aggression', *Journal of Communication,* 28 (3): 12–29.

Bauman, Zygmunt (2010): 'Media, Bystanders, Actors', *Responsibility in Context* (Springer): 95–101.

Beech, Bernard, and Phil Leather(2006): 'Workplace violence in the health care sector: A review of staff training and integration of training evaluation models', *Aggression and Violent Behavior,* 11 (1): 27–43.

Bies, Robert J., and Thomas M. Tripp (1996): 'Beyond Distrust: "Getting Even" and the Need for Revenge', (Chapter 12 of book titled 'Trust in Organizations: Frontiers of Theory and Research', United Kingdom, Sage).

Bowlby, John (2005): *A Secure Base: Clinical applications of attachment theory* (United Kingdom, Taylor & Francis).

Campbell, Anne (1995): 'A few good men: Evolutionary psychology and female adolescent aggression', *Ethology and Sociobiology*, 16 (2): 99–123.

Campbell, Anne (1999): 'The last days of discord? Evolution and culture as accounts of female-female aggression', *Behavioral and Brain Sciences*, 22 (02): 237–46.

Clegg, Stewart R. (1993), 'Narrative, Power and Social Theory', (Chapter 1 in *Narrative and Social Control: Critical Perspectives*, United Kingdom, Sage).

Collins, Randall (2009): 'Micro and macro causes of violence', *International Journal of Conflict and Violence (IJCV)*, 3 (1): 9–22.

Cooper, Laurie Ball, et al. (2013): 'Reducing gender-based violence', *The Sage Handbook of Gender and Psychology* (London, UK: Sage).

Dollard, John, et al. (1939), 'Frustration and Aggression'. (New Haven, CT, US, Yale University Press).

Donabedian, Avedis (1988): 'The quality of care: How can it be assessed?', *Jama*, 260 (12): 1743–8.

Donabedian, Avedis (2005): 'Evaluating the quality of medical care', *Milbank Quarterly*, 83 (4): 691–729.

Eagly, Alice H., and Valerie J. Steffen (1986): 'Gender and aggressive behavior: A meta-analytic review of the social psychological literature', *Psychological Bulletin*, 100 (3): 309.

Eagly, Alice H., et al. (2000): 'Social role theory of sex differences and similarities: A current appraisal', *Developmental Social Psychology of Gender*: 123–74.

Einarsen, Stale, and Anders Skogstad (1996): 'Bullying at work:

Epidemiological findings in public and private organizations', *European Journal of Work and Organizational Psychology,* 5 (2): 185–201.

Eisenhardt, Kathleen M. (1989): 'Agency theory: An assessment and review', *Academy of Management Review,* 14 (1): 57–74.

Estabrooks, Carole A., et al. (2006): 'A guide to knowledge translation theory', *Journal of Continuing Education in the Health Professions,* 26 (1): 25–36.

Fitzgerald, Louise F., and Alayne J. Ormerod (1993): 'Breaking silence: The sexual harassment of women in academia and the workplace', (Chapter in *Psychology of women: A handbook of issues and theories,* Westport, CT, US: Greenwood Press/Greenwood Publishing Group).

Freud, Sigmund (1967): *Moses and Monotheism,* translated by Katherine Jones (New York: Vintage Books).

Freud, Sigmund (1918): 'Totem and taboo, translation by A.A. Brill, (New York: Moffat, Yard & Co).

Freud, Sigmund (1930): *Civilization and its Discontents,* translated by James Strachey (New York, W.W. Norton and Company).

Gastaldo, Denise, and Dave Holmes(1999): 'Foucault and nursing: A history of the present', *Nursing Inquiry,* 6 (4): 231–40.

Hartsock, Nancy (1990): 'Foucault on power: A theory for women?', *Feminism/Postmodernism:* 162.

Hesketh, Kathryn L., et al. (2003): 'Workplace violence in Alberta and British Columbia hospitals', *Health Policy,* 63 (3): 311–21.

Hogg, Michael A. (2006): 'Social Identity Theory', *Contemporary Social Psychological Theories,* 13: 111–369.

Huskinson, Lucy (2002): 'The self as violent other: The problem of defining the self', *Journal of Analytical Psychology,* 47 (3): 437–58.

Hussain, Rafat, and Adeel Khan (2008): 'Women's perceptions and experiences of sexual violence in marital relationships and its effect on reproductive health', *Health Care for Women International*, 29 (5): 468–83.

Hutchinson, Marie, et al. (2006): 'Workplace bullying in nursing: towards a more critical organisational perspective', *Nursing Inquiry*, 13 (2): 118–26.

Islam, Nasir (2004): 'Sifarish, sycophants, power and collectivism: administrative culture in Pakistan', *International Review of Administrative Sciences*, 70 (2): 311–30.

Kanter Moss, Rosabeth (1977): 'Men and Women of the Corporation', (New York: Basic Books).

Kuumba, Monica Bahati (1994): 'The Limits of Feminism: Decolonizing Women's Liberation/Oppression Theory', *Race, Sex & Class*: 85–100.

Larwood, Laurie, and Marion M. Wood, M. (1977): 'Women in Management' (United States: Lexington Books).

Laschinger, Heather K. Spence, et al. (2000): 'Organizational trust and empowerment in restructured healthcare settings: effects on staff nurse commitment', *Journal of Nursing Administration*, 30 (9): 413–25.

Leininger, Madeleine, and Marilyn R. McFarland (2002): 'Transcultural Nursing: Concepts, theories, research and practice', *Journal of Transcultural Nursing*, 13 (3): 261.

Lew, Amy, and Betty Lou Bettner (2002): *A parent's guide to understanding and motivating children* (United States, Connexions Press).

Lincoln, James R., and Didier Guillot (2004): 'Durkheim and organizational culture', *Institute for Research on Labor and Employment* (IRLE) Working Paper, Berkeley.

Mack, D.A., et al. (1998): 'Stress and the preventative management of workplace violence', *Monographs in Organizational Behavior and Industrial Relations*, 23: 119–42.

MacKinnon, Catharine A. (1979): *Sexual harassment of working women: A case of sex discrimination* (New Haven: Yale University Press).

Martinko, Mark J., and William L. Gardner (1982): 'Learned helplessness: An alternative explanation for performance deficits', *Academy of Management Review,* 7 (2): 195–204.

Megargee, Edwin I (1966): 'Undercontrolled and overcontrolled personality types in extreme antisocial aggression', *Psychological Monographs: General and Applied,* 80 (3): 1.

O'Leary-Kelly, Anne M., et al. (1996): 'Organization-motivated aggression: A research framework', *Academy of Management Review,* 21 (1): 225–53.

Ones, Deniz S.,et al. (1993): 'Comprehensive meta-analysis of integrity test validities: Findings and implications for personnel selection and theories of job performance', *Journal of Applied Psychology,* 78 (4): 679.

Reeves, Scott, et al. (2008): 'Why use theories in qualitative research', *BMJ,* 337 (7670): 631–34.

Schafer, Stephen (1967): *The Victim and His Criminal: Victimology* (United States, President's Commission on Law Enforcement and Administration of Justice).

Spector, Paul E. (1982): 'Behavior in organizations as a function of employee's locus of control', *Psychological Bulletin,* 91 (3): 482.

Strauss, Anselm, et al. (1963): 'The hospital and its negotiated order' in Eliot Friedson, ed. *The Hospital in Modern* Society (New York: Free Press of Glencoe.

Taylor, Shelley E. (1983): 'Adjustment to threatening events: A theory of cognitive adaptation', *American Psychologist,* 38 (11): 1161.

Thau, Stefan, et al. (2009): 'How management style moderates the relationship between abusive supervision and workplace deviance: An uncertainty management theory perspective', *Organizational Behavior and Human Decision Processes,* 108 (1): 79–92.

Toch, Hans (1993): 'Good violence and bad violence: Through self-presentations of aggressors accounts and war stories', (Chapter in *Aggression and violence: Social interactionist perspectives*, Washington, DC, US: American Psychological Association).

Vaughan, Diane (2004): 'Theorizing Disaster Analogy, Historical Ethnography, and the Challenger Accident', *Ethnography*, 5 (3): 315–47.

Walton, Gerald (2005): 'The notion of bullying through the lens of Foucault and critical theory', *Journal of Educational Thought (JET)/Revue de la Pensée Educative*: 55–73.

Watson, David, Lee A. Clark, and Auke Tellegen (1988): 'Development and validation of brief measures of positive and negative affect: the PANAS scales', *Journal of Personality and Social Psychology*, 54 (6): 1063.

Willetts, Georgina, and David Clarke (2014): 'Constructing nurses' professional identity through social identity theory', *International Journal of Nursing Practice*, 20 (2): 164–9.

Williams, Philippa, et al. (2004): 'Defining social support in context: A necessary step in improving research, intervention, and practice', *Qualitative Health Research*, 14 (7): 942–60.

Wilson, James Q. and Kelling, George L. Kelling (1982): 'Broken windows', *Critical Issues in Policing: Contemporary Readings*: 395–407.

## NOTES

1. Co-workers of nurses in the health sector include other nurses, physicians, surgeons, administrators, therapists, paramedical staff, and pharmacists.
2. Inequalities begin to widen and oppressed groups, especially women, systematically lose power and privilege. Since stratification is culturally accepted, oppressed groups assume low professional status.
3. Mechanical solidarity refers to the necessary collaboration between

different members of society who are dependent on each other due to common beliefs and practices. It was a term used by Emile Durkheim (1858–1917) to depict collective conscience which helped to promote solidarity and cooperation through division of labour and interdependent work.

4. The documentation of a patient's ongoing treatment is strongly controlled by power relations within the hospital setting and across wider community. For example, a woman practitioner with less power and status would be less able to communicate diagnosis and mobilize co-worker support for alternative treatment that could save a patient's life.

5. The different principal groups for women healthcare practitioners include ward supervisors, departmental heads, administrators, clinical instructors, and senior doctors and surgeons at the hospital.

# 3

# Quantitative Evidence of Workplace Violence

To add value to previous scholarship and dispel ambiguities, it became important to collect more data about the realities of workplace violence against women healthcare practitioners in Pakistan. As an academician, the major concern for me was the decision to resolve in practical terms the questions arising from the philosophical background to my research. The realist researcher believes in foundationalist ontology which theorizes that gender inequality does exists in society but also highlights that direct observation cannot unlock deeply-layered structural relationships (Olsen 2004). In order to understand structure, it becomes important also to comprehend the beliefs and attitudes that control an organization. Therefore it seems prudent to simultaneously investigate action with structure as concurrent forces influencing processes and outcomes (Giddens 1979). That is why I decided to take a realist research approach and adopt a mixed methods model to derive the benefits of both methodological pluralism and triangulation (Plowright 2011). The quantitative data was collected with the help of an internationally validated tool during the period between November 2015 and January 2016 (ILO/ICN/WHO/PSI 2003). The aim has been to ascertain statistical prevalence and also to unlock hidden socio-cultural

73

and region-specific narratives about perceived causes and precipitators of workplace violence.

## Types of Women Healthcare Practitioners in Pakistan

Women traditional birth attendants (TBAs) played a crucial role in supporting women and children of South Asia in the past but they lacked skill and training and thus compromised the lives of women and children (Aftab 2007). In lieu of this, the lady health workers programme was launched by the government of Pakistan in 1994 to facilitate family planning and primary healthcare for disadvantaged women across rural and less developed urban areas of the country. A total of 110,000 LHWs have been trained through the programme to provide health support to community women at their doorsteps. Healthcare units, which serve as the official base for LHWs, are operational in every city, *tehsil* or sub-district, and village of Pakistan. LHWs provide preventive, minor curative, referral, and rehabilitative services to the community. On average, up to 25 LHWs report to one lady health supervisor (LHS), and up to 50 LHSs report to one district health officer. However, the specialized services of LHWs for family planning, reproductive health, immunization, and abortion-care have been extremely resented by conservative communities. Many believe that LHWs have been funded and trained by Western agencies to ruin the health of their women and children, and this has led to critical rates of violence against them (Ayub & Siddiqui 2013).

An estimated 7,86,000 nurses are licensed to practise in the country by the Pakistan Nursing Council (PNC), of which over 95 per cent are women. However, the nurse to doctor and nurse to patient ratios are below the internationally recommended rates (World Health Organization 2005). There is only one nurse for every three doctors, and only one nurse for up to 50,000 patients. This is a dire shortfall if one considers that the average number of patients in a public sector hospital general ward is 50, and that if more than one has an emergency at the same time, they will remain unattended due to nurse shortages. Additionally, one nurse is being used to execute the orders of three doctors at a time, when international standards require that three nurses should be supporting one doctor as a feasible ratio for patient safety. Invariably, nurse shortage and high work burdens contribute to sustained violence against nurses. Due to the acute organizational problems and high rate of violence, fewer women in Pakistan want to enter the nursing profession.

There are a total of 80,562 women doctors in Pakistan, among which 10,005 are dentists. Despite high enrolment of women in medical schools, their participation as practitioners in healthcare delivery is nearly half that of the list of medical graduates (Rehman et al. 2011). This is because, although medical degrees hold high status for women, practising the profession cancels the high status afforded to the female medical graduate. Also, interaction with non-blood male relatives is frowned upon and stigmatized as a consequence of religious and cultural beliefs. The women who do practice medicine remain in the less influential and feminized specializations of pathology, paediatrics, gynaecology, and family practice. Some choose to teach in women medical colleges, while others bow to the social pressures to get married and become housewives. Not only are there many fewer women doctors in comparison to their male counterparts but they have little control over governance and policymaking. Women doctors will not be found as elected or assigned representatives of health bodies such as the Pakistan Medical and Dental Council (PMDC), Pakistan Healthcare Commission, or the Ministry of National Health Services. In general, women doctors in Pakistan have remained characteristically submissive and this has prevented them from asserting their rights, equality, and safety (Arif 2011). It is this compliant and non-aggressive identity of theirs which contributes to bullying, harassment, and overall violence against them.

## The Condition of Public Hospitals in Pakistan

Hospitals are complex organizations comprising of a large number of specialists working together in diverse and interdependent operations, with immense pressure to save lives (Lok & Crawford 1999). The three principal features of hospital organizational culture are: (1) it is socially constructed by groups based on shared experiences, (2) it is specific and unique to every society, and (3) it is not rigid or fixed over time (Bellot 2011). Lack of resource allocation, equitable investment, and ineffective policy decisions have become a cause of major concern for Pakistan's health sector (Akram & Khan 2007). Reports and analytical recommendations for improvement of practitioner services and organizational culture are available but implementation and enforcement is lacking across Pakistan (Nishtar 2006). The most alarming problem is the regular and sustained abuse against women practitioners (d'Oliveira et al. 2002). A study by Saeed and Ibrahim (2005) assessed doctor views at a tertiary-care public sector hospital in order to confirm the main problems faced by healthcare employees and patients. The interviews revealed critical problem areas, such as: inadequate pay and promotions, shortages of staff, absence of a clinical orientation for new graduates and training opportunities for old staff, and a lack of supervision and regulatory bodies. Nearly all the doctors described their insecurity at the workplace given the frequent and unrelenting violence suffered at the hands of patients and family attendants.

Reports have emphasized that women healthcare practitioners are dissatisfied with their career development, salary structures, and the available educational infrastructure (Gulzar et al. 2010). Job satisfaction and career development is compromised due to an absence of a supportive teaching faculty and a learning-based culture (Bahalkani et al. 2011). Researchers have assessed the problems women practitioners encounter in fulfilling their maternal roles given the absence of organizational support from the healthcare administration (Zafar & Bustamante-Gavino 2008). The findings draw attention to the absence of quality day care centres or private rooms for expressing and storing milk of lactating mothers during work hours. The studies, though few, have been significant in highlighting the absence of structural support for women practitioners and their ability to control workplace benefits and employee policies.

Women healthcare practitioners have serious communication problems during role delivery in the hospital setting (Azhar et al. 2009). There is a sustained lack of support and unmet expectations from co-workers which contributes to women providers' inefficiency in role delivery. Critical issues of drug-related problems and medical errors are being caused by a lack of collaboration between healthcare professionals. The failed links between dependent specialists in the healthcare sector has its roots in the common disrespect and low status allocated to women practitioners.

The public sector hospitals in Pakistan have weak patient-safety standards and there are no error-tracking systems in place. They also suffer from a punitive blame culture against individual women who are found to commit or report errors. There have been no formal efforts within hospital organizations or by the health sector to educate professionals and the public about non-punitive actions taken against practitioners when errors occur. In addition, there has been limited medical curriculum inclusion, on-the-job training, and policy guidelines on how to deal with errors at the workplace. Indeed, managers and supervisors have been known to teach novice practitioners, through the hidden curriculum, not to report errors because they do not harm the patient (Kingston et al. 2004). Given the cultural attitudes towards women practitioners, more blame is placed on them when errors occur in the hospital setting (Hashemi et al. 2012). Undoubtedly, when women healthcare practitioners make more errors at the workplace, the rate of aggression and violence against them increases (Kamchuchat et al. 2008).

# Findings

## Socio-demographics and prevalence of workplace violence

The socio-demographic results of the sample reflect the actual weightage of women healthcare practitioners across Pakistan but the results must still be interpreted with caution when generalizations are made, which is true for any empirical study. As shown in Table 1, the Chi-squared results are highly significant with regard to the socio-demographic variables of women healthcare practitioners for all three types of violence. The mean age of the sample is 32 years, with the minimum and maximum ages of women falling between 20 to 66 years. Nearly half the women, at 47 per cent, are between the ages of 20–29, and 37 per cent are between the ages of 30–39. Most of the women in the sample are of a younger demographic which matches the working population statistics presented by the Pakistan Economic Survey 2015–16. International scholarship suggests that younger women are at a greater risk of facing all manner of violence, especially sexual violence (Watts & Zimmerman 2002). Chi-squared results show that physical violence ($X^2$= 35.706, p<.001), verbal violence ($X^2$= 13.160, p<.05), and sexual violence ($X^2$= 18.953, p<.001) are significantly associated with the age of the women practitioners.

Nearly half the sample, at 44 per cent, is not married, and 56 per cent is either currently married or has been married. Of the married women, a majority at 55 per cent have 3 to 6 children, while 39 per cent have children below the age of 2 years. Chi-squared results show that physical violence ($X^2$= 23.165, p<.001), verbal violence ($X^2$= 3.933, p<.05), and sexual violence ($X^2$= 5.710, p<.05) are significantly associated with the marital status of women practitioners. It is important to consider here that the prevalent statistics for violence against married women may be under-reported because married working women in Pakistan are under great pressure to return home and resume household responsibilities which means they have less time to seek accountability against verbal violence or less impactful violence such as minor physical assault. Besides, married women with children are less comfortable reporting the experience of violence, especially sexual violence, as this might cause problems in their marriage or their relationship with their in-laws, and may also lead to doubts or slander about their children's legitimacy. Expectedly, single women would be even less willing to report violence due to fears of family dishonour.

Most of the women respondents are from the province of Punjab (Lahore, Islamabad, Rawalpindi, other cities in Punjab), at 52 per cent, and Sindh (Karachi), at 47 per cent. Women respondents indicated that they had experienced significant levels of all types of violence in all the three cities of Karachi (capital city of Sindh), Lahore (capital city of Punjab), and Islamabad (capital of Pakistan/city in Punjab province). A range of cities from Punjab have been sampled including Sargodha, Sheikhupura, Rajanpur, Jaranwala, Gujranwala, Faisalabad, Sialkot, Kasur, Kamlia, Rawalpindi, and Sahiwal. Chi square results show that physical violence ($X^2$= 15.360, p<.05), verbal violence ($X^2$= 19.672, p<.05), and sexual violence ($X^2$= 24.637, p<.05), are significantly associated with all the cities sampled. Workplace violence in Pakistan seems to be a countrywide norm, regardless of the province or city, lending strength to the argument that violence is condoned by socio-structural and legislative failure across Pakistan.

The mean income per month for sampled women practitioners overall is PKR 29,335, with minimum wages for LHWs at PKR 5,000 and maximum wages for a few senior doctors at PKR 100,000. Nearly half of the sampled women (47 per cent) earn a monthly income between PKR 20,000 and 39,000. Regrettably, this income bracket and the mean income are below the average salary for professionals in Pakistan. Chi-squared results show that physical violence ($X^2$= 12.581, p<.005), verbal violence ($X^2$= 1.882, p<.05), and sexual violence ($X^2$= 21.970, p<.001) are significantly associated with the level of income earned. It may be that underpaid women employees in the Pakistani healthcare sector face more horizontal and verbal violence from their male colleagues, seniors, and administration because income levels have a correlation with status and rank. Perpetrator co-workers begin to believe that if women have been unable to lobby for equal pay and compensation in the past, they will be unable to fight for retribution against assailants in the future.

Nearly all women healthcare practitioners (93 per cent) live in private accommodation not provided by the government, and the same percentage (93 per cent) work full-time at their respective workplaces. Notwithstanding full-time employment, 14 per cent of women indicated that they work in private clinics in their spare time. Private employment suggests that there is pressure on some women healthcare practitioners who have to solely, or largely, contribute to household expenses and simultaneously sustain two jobs in order to combat rising economic costs and inflation. Chi-squared results show that physical violence ($X^2$= 5.549, p<.05) and verbal violence ($X^2$= 14.574, p<.001) are significantly associated with the place of residence of women practitioners. It may be that women in hospital-provided accommodation are at a greater risk of violence, especially when they are living alone without a male guardian and also because employee residences can be easily traced by co-workers and in-patients on the basis of hospital records.

Nearly 70 per cent of the employees are on a permanent contract of which 61 per cent of these are from a 16 or 17 government grade. Interestingly, although a government employee rank should deter patients and attendants from wreaking violence against women healthcare practitioners, this is not the case in Pakistan. Chi-square results indicate that physical violence ($X^2$= 9.000, p<.05) and verbal violence ($X^2$= 4.727, p<.05) are significantly associated with the permanency of the women practitioners' contract. Women practitioners on permanent contract face violence as a consequence of weak accountability structures and the confidence of the perpetrators that government jobs are incapable of securing justice for women employees. Similarly, contractual women employees also face violence because they enjoy even less structural support when reporting and seeking retribution against the perpetrators. It is relevant too that contractual women employees who are awaiting recommendations for a permanent contract, would also be less inclined to report violence. Chi-squared results show that physical violence ($X^2$= 9.033, p<.05), verbal violence ($X^2$= 2.325, p<.05), and sexual violence ($X^2$= 14.524, p<.005) are significantly associated with the government grade of women practitioners. It is understandable again that government rank does not deter perpetrators from perpetrating violence against women practitioners, as women government officers are believed to have fewer professional affiliations that provide assistance in justice.

A total of 74 per cent of the women respondents mentioned having to work additional hours after shift time and 52 per cent are obliged to undertake compulsory night duties. The Chi-square results show that: (1) physical violence ($X^2$= 6.143, p<.05), verbal violence ($X^2$= 2.430, p<.5), and sexual violence ($X^2$= 3.553, p<.5) are significantly associated with working additional hours and that, (2) physical violence ($X^2$= 10.797, p<.001) and verbal violence ($X^2$= 2.170, p<.05) are significantly associated with night duties. Working extra hours and especially undertaking night duty is known to place women healthcare practitioners at a higher risk of violence given the absence of a considerable proportion of staff and outpatients during these time slots.

## Table 1

Frequency and chi square results for violence experienced by women healthcare practitioners in Pakistan according to socio-demographic characteristics.

|  | Total f (%) | Experi-enced PV f (%) | Experi-enced VV f (%) | Experi-enced SV f (%) |
|---|---|---|---|---|
| **Age in years** | | | | |
| 20–29 | 188 (46.9) | 43 (22.9) | 128 (68.1) | 73 (31.0) |
| 30–39 | 149 (37.2) | 79 (53.0) | 121 (81.2) | 63 (42.3) |
| 40–49 | 40 (10.0) | 20 (50.0) | 34 (85.0) | 24 (60.0) |
| 50+ | 24 (05.9) | 09 (39.1) | 16 (69.6) | – |
| Chi square | | 35.706 | 13.160 | 18.953 |
| significance, p value | | <0.001 | <0.05 | <0.001 |
| **Marital Status** | | | | |
| Never married | 177 (44.1) | 48 (27.1) | 127 (71.8) | 65 (36.7) |
| Currently married | 202 (50.4) | 99 (49.0) | 152 (75.2) | 82 (40.8) |
| Widowed/divorced/separated | 22 (05.4) | 04 (19.0) | 20 (95.2) | 13 (61.9) |
| | | 23.165 | 3.933 | 5.710 |
| Chi-square significance, p value | | <0.001 | <0.5 | <0.5 |
| **Region** | | | | |
| Lahore | 146 (36.4) | 55 (36.4) | 106 (35.5) | 73 (24.4) |
| Other cities of Punjab | 21 (04.5) | 10 (04.6) | 13 (03.3) | 09 (02.3) |
| Karachi, | 190 (47.4) | 72 (47.7) | 148 (49.5) | 62 (20.7) |
| Islamabad, Rawalpindi | 44 (11.0) | 14 (9.3) | 32 (10.7) | 16 (05.4) |
| Chi-square significance, p value | | 15.360 <0.5 | 19.672 <0.5 | 24.637 <0.05 |
| **Religion** | | | | |
| Muslim | 323 (80.5) | 114 (35.3) | 239 (75.0) | 128 (39.6) |
| Christian | 76 (19.0) | 36 (47.4) | 59 (77.6) | 31 (41.3) |
| Hindu | 02 (0.5) | 01 (50) | 01 (50) | 01 (50) |
| Chi-square significance, p value | | 3.951 <0.5 | 1.069 0.586/N.S | 0.157 0.924/N.S. |

| | Total f (%) | Experi-enced PV f (%) | Experi-enced VV f (%) | Experi-enced SV f (%) |
|---|---|---|---|---|
| **Children** | | | | |
| 1–2 | 70 (38.7) | 34 (37.0) | 63 (43.4) | 25 (30.9) |
| 3–6 | 100 (55.2) | 52 (56.5) | 73 (50.3) | 52 (64.2) |
| ≥ 6 | 11 (06.1) | 06 (06.5) | 09 (6.2) | 04 (04.9) |
| Chi-square significance, p value | | 3.202 0.524/N.S | 8.430 <0.5 | 3.610 <0.5 |
| **Age of last child** | | | | |
| Less than 1 year | 10 (05.5) | 07 (70.0) | 08 (80.0) | 04 (40.0) |
| 1–5 years | 74 (40.3) | 42 (56.8) | 64 (86.5) | 31 (41.9) |
| 6 years and above | 98 (54.1) | 43 (43.9) | 74 (75.5) | 47 (48.0) |
| Chi-square significance, p value | | 4.399 <0.5 | 3.202 <0.5 | 0.736 0.692/N.S. |
| **Income** | | | | |
| ≤19,999 | 117 (29.2) | 49 (45.4) | 83 (76.9) | 31 (28.7) |
| 20,000–39,999 | 180 (47.1) | 54 (28.6) | 135 (71.4) | 68 (36.2) |
| ≥ 40,000 | 104 (25.9) | 48 (46.2) | 81 (77.9) | 61 (58.7) |
| Chi-square significance, p value | | 12.581 <0.005 | 1.882 <0.5 | 21.970 <0.001 |
| **Residence** | | | | |
| Hospital-provided | 29 (07.2) | 05 (17.2) | 13 (44.8) | 10 (34.5) |
| Private | 372 (92.8) | 146 (39.2) | 286 (76.9) | 150 (40.4) |
| Chi-square significance, p value | | 5.549 <0.05 | 14.574 <0.001 | 0.397 0.529/N.S. |
| **Government Contract** | 123 (30.7) | 33 (26.8) | 84 (68.3) | 48 (39.0) |
| Contractual Permanent | 278 (69.3) | 118 (42.4) | 215 (77.3) | 112 (40.3) |
| Chi-square significance, p value | | 9.000 <0.05 | 4.727 <0.5 | 0.101 0.951/N.S. |
| **Employment Status** | | | | |
| Full-time | 373 (93.0) | 144 (38.6) | 280 (75.1) | 146 (39.1) |
| Part-time | 28 (07.0) | 07 (25.0) | 19 (67.9) | 14 (50.0) |
| Chi-square significance, p value | | 2.097 <0.5 | 1.772 <0.5 | 5.519 <0.5 |

| | Total f (%) | Experi-enced PV f (%) | Experi-enced VV f (%) | Experi-enced SV f (%) |
|---|---|---|---|---|
| **Government Grade** | | | | |
| 16 grade | 129 (32.2) | 58 (45.0) | 100 (77.5) | 67 (51.9) |
| 17 grade | 115 (28.7) | 31 (27.0) | 81 (70.4) | 42 (36.8) |
| 18 grade | 13 (03.2) | 06 (46.2) | 11 (84.6) | 07 (53.8) |
| Other (contractual or LHW) | 144 (35.9) | 56 (38.9) | 107 (74.3) | 44 (30.6) |
| | | 9.033 | 2.325 | 14.524 |
| Chi-square significance, p value | | <0.05 | <0.5 | <0.005 |
| **Employed at private clinic** | 54 (13.5) | 26 (48.1) | 42 (77.8) | 35 (64.8) |
| Yes | 347 (86.5) | 125 (36.0) | 257 (74.1) | 125 (36.1) |
| No | | | | |
| | | 2.926 | 0.340 | 16.017 |
| Chi-square significance, p value | | <0.5 | 0.560/N.S. | <0.001 |
| **Additional working hours after shift time** | 296 (73.8) | 102 (34.5) | 215 (72.6) | 111 (37.6) |
| Yes | 105 (26.1) | 49 (46.2) | 84 (79.8) | 49 (47.1) |
| No | | | | |
| | | 6.143 | 2.430 | 3.553 |
| Chi-square significance, p value | | <0.05 | <0.5 | <0.5 |
| **Have to work night shifts** | 210 (52.4) | 95 (45.2) | 163 (77.6) | 88 (41.9) |
| Yes | 191 (47.6) | 56 (29.3) | 136 (71.2) | 72 (37.9) |
| No | | | | |
| | | 10.797 | 2.170 | 0.668 |
| Chi-square significance, p value | | 0.001 | <0.5 | 0.414 |
| **Total** | 401 (100%) | 151 (37.7%) | 299 (74.6%) | 158 (39.4%) |

Key: PV: Physical Violence, VV: Verbal Violence, SV: Sexual Violence

## Workplace violence across hospitals and Basic Health Units

The tertiary-care public sector hospitals in urban cities like Lahore, Karachi, and Islamabad are mostly frequented by a majority of the poor and illiterate patients. This is primarily because of the ease of access and rate concessions. However, due to low fund allocations for the health sector, amounting to under 2 per cent of the government budget, the organizational culture is extremely inefficient and well below international standards. Unequipped buildings, resource and staffing shortages, and unmet health demands generate insecurity and aggression amongst the public. In addition, there are no formal or informal systems in place to secure the safety of women practitioners or women patients in Pakistan's public hospitals.

I have been through the process of interviewing women nurses from public sector hospitals during my doctoral research, and thus revisiting hospitals to interview women nurses and doctors was largely unproblematic. Permissions to collect data have to be taken from different supervisors, depending upon the hospital policy, which included hospital principals, medical superintendents, heads of departments and wards, nurse principals, and nurse supervisors. Approaching LHWs broadened my research to include basic health units (BHUs) or family welfare centres, which took more time and required permission from the directors of the Punjab and Sindh Healthcare Departments. LHWs were the most approachable and willing participants during my data collection experience. Many expressed happiness that research was being undertaken into the violence they faced and many also remarked that they were eager to hear that my findings were being communicated to relevant bodies who could affect improvements in terms of their safety and development. LHWs completed their surveys at BHUs, while doctors and nurses completed theirs in rooms reserved in the wards or the nursing schools of the respective hospitals. I or my research assistants were present to resolve any ambiguity or confusion raised by the survey questions.

The internationally standardized instrument evolved by the World Health Organization was employed to measure workplace violence against healthcare providers and ensure the validity and reliability of the research. The survey was shortened to include only those questions that are relevant to practitioners working in the public health sector of Pakistan and so that the final 39 questions were not too taxing for busy women practitioners. Violence was described to respondents in terms of any assault or abuse which included physical assault, homicide, verbal abuse, bullying or mobbing, sexual and racial harassment, or psychological stress. Participants were reminded that violence does not only occur as one single incident but might also be expressed in terms of repeated small incidents which together constitute grievous harm.

As was to be expected, the women practitioners, especially the doctors, were extremely hesitant to answer questions about experiencing violence at the workplace. I had to overcome the reluctance in prospective participants by investing time during the pre-interview and research communication phase. Ward heads and my research assistants were instrumental in providing support during this time. It was communicated to prospective participants, through meetings and in a written introductory cover letter, that: (1) their contribution was important in ascertaining statistics for the prevalence of workplace violence and understanding perceived causes, (2) their responses would not be traced back to them, (3) a considerable number of working women were facing violence in Pakistan and it constituted a dangerous reality which had been ignored for too long, and (4) women from the developed world had secured rights and safety for themselves at the workplace through disclosure and research participation.

A total of 401 women practitioners were sampled from the national capital, Islamabad, and the provincial capitals of Punjab and Sindh, (the cities of Lahore and Karachi respectively).[1] It was not possible to collect data from other provinces, like Balochistan and KPK, due to security concerns for women researchers and permission problems. It is also noteworthy that a larger number of public sector hospitals exist in Punjab and Sindh given their greater population count and higher budget allocations in comparison to the other provinces. Data was collected from 11 public sector hospitals[2], as presented in Table 2, which included: (1) From Lahore: Jinnah Hospital, Lahore; Sheikh Zayed Hospital, Mayo Hospital, Ganga Ram Hospital, INMOL, and United Christian Hospital; (2) From Karachi: Jinnah Hospital, Karachi; Civil Hospital, Sindh; Government Health Department, and Pakistan Naval Society, Rahat, and (3) From Islamabad: Pakistan Institute of Medical Sciences (PIMS). All these are large tertiary-care public sector hospitals, offering almost free healthcare services with exhaustive medical and surgical departments and including 24-hour emergency services. Each of them have a large turnover averaging somewhere between 1,000 patients a day and 1,000 in-patient bed capacities. The following public hospitals that were sampled have affiliated medical and nursing colleges, including Jinnah Hospital (Lahore), Sheikh Zayed, Mayo, Ganga Ram, Jinnah Hospital (Karachi), and Civil Hospital (Karachi). Eight BHUs[3] were sampled to access LHWs in the localities of: (1) Baghban Pura/Shalimar, and Shahdra in Lahore; (2) Shanti Nagar, Pehlwan Goth, Gharibabad,

Hussain Hazara, and PIB Maternity Home in Karachi; and (3) Saddar in Rawalpindi.

Women practitioners across hospitals and BHUs faced physical violence between ranges of 4 to 100 per cent, verbal violence between 21 to 100 per cent, and sexual violence ranging from 2 to 83 per cent. Chi-square results show highly significant levels of physical violence ($X^2$= 57.957, p<.001), verbal violence ($X^2$= 98.607, p<.001), and sexual violence ($X^2$= 26.517, p<.05) faced by women practitioners across all workplaces. Results show that regardless of whether it was a hospital or a BHU, women practitioners face all types of violence as a hazardous reality at their place of work. For the women of Pakistan, the prevalent patriarchal and gender discriminatory society are replicated in the internal structures of all public hospitals. The parlous state of public hospitals in Pakistan, with their current structural shortcomings and high rates of violence against women employees who are integral to their functioning, is a testimony to the competence and resilience of women practitioners.

Table 2

Frequency and chi-squared results for violence experienced by women healthcare practitioners in Pakistan according to hospital or basic health unit.

|  | Total $f$ (%) | Experienced PV $f$ (%) | Experienced VV $f$ (%) | Experienced SV $f$ (%) |
|---|---|---|---|---|
| **Lahore** |  |  |  |  |
| Jinnah Hospital, Lahore | 67 (16.7) | 29 (43.3) | 54 (80.6) | 30 (44.8) |
| Sheikh Zayed Hospital | 39 (09.7) | 13 (33.3) | 28 (71.8) | 22 (56.4) |
| INMOL Hospital | 26 (06.5) | 10 (38.5) | 22 (84.6) | 12 (46.2) |

| | Total f (%) | Experienced PV f (%) | Experienced VV f (%) | Experienced SV f (%) |
|---|---|---|---|---|
| United Christian Hospital, Lahore | 26 (06.5) | 10 (38.5) | 22 (84.6) | 09 (34.6) |
| Mayo Hospital | 25 (06.2) | 05 (20.0) | 13 (52.5) | 06 (24.0) |
| Ganga Ram Hospital | 24 (06.0) | 01 (04.2) | 05 (20.8) | 01 (04.2) |
| Baghban Pura BHU/ Shalimar BHU | 10 (02.5) | 06 (60.0) | 07 (70.0) | 07 (70.0) |
| Shahdra BHU | 02 (00.5) | 01 (50.0) | 02 (100.0) | 01 (50.0) |
| **Karachi** | | | | |
| Jinnah Hospital, Karachi | 56 (14.0) | 25 (44.6) | 42 (75.0) | 01 (01.8) |
| Civil Hospital, Karachi | 42 (10.5) | 13 (31.0) | 32 (76.2) | 18 (42.9) |
| Sindh Government Health Department | 33 (08.2) | 03 (09.1) | 08 (24.2) | 02 (06.1) |
| Pakistan Naval Society, Rahat | 20 (05.0) | 05 (25.0) | 05 (25.0) | 01 (05.0) |
| Pehlwan Goth BHU | 06 (01.5) | 06 (100.0) | 06 (100.0) | 05 (83.0) |
| Gharibabad Dispensary | 04 (01.0) | 04 (100.0) | 04 (100.0) | 02 (50.0) |
| Hussain Hazara BHU | 04 (01.0) | 03 (75.0) | 04 (100.0) | 02 (50.0) |
| PIB Maternity Home, | 03 (00.7) | 02 (66.7) | 03 (100.0) | 02 (66.7) |
| Shanti Nagar Dispensary | 03 (00.7) | 01 (33.3) | 03 (100.0) | 01 (33.3) |
| **Islamabad/ Rawalpindi** | | | | |
| Pakistan Institute of Medical Sciences | 43 (10.7) | 14 (32.6) | 32 (74.4) | 28 (65.1) |
| Saddar BHU | 17 (04.2) | 02 (11.8) | 07 (41.2) | 05 (29.4) |
| Chi-square Significance, p value | | 57.957 <0.001 | 98.607 <0.001 | 26.517 <0.05 |
| **Total** | 401 (100%) | 151 (37.7%) | 299 (74.6%) | 160 (39.9%) |
| **Key**: PV: Physical Violence, VV: Verbal Violence, SV: Sexual Violence | | | | |

## *Workplace violence across degrees, departments, and designations*

The prevalence and significance of workplace violence was investigated according to the academic qualifications of the women practitioners concerned, as set out in Table 3. A total of 112 women doctors and 41 dentists were sampled, as set out in Table 2. Most (N=94) of the doctors had qualified for the MBBS (Bachelor of Medicine, Bachelor of Surgery), and some (N=18) had further specialized with an FCPS (Fellowship of the College of Physicians and Surgeons) or a PhD in public health. Regardless of the level of academic qualification of the women doctors, all of them indicated that they had experienced all types of violence at the workplace, with physical violence indicated in the range between 18 to 50 per cent, verbal violence between 56 and 100 per cent, and sexual violence between 18 and 50 per cent. When interpreting these figures, we must bear in mind that for high status degree holders, like women doctors who might also belong to a higher socio-economic class, it would be self-defamatory to admit to having experienced violence, even confidentially and in a written survey. This is because medicine as a profession has been accorded a high cultural status and it means a loss of honour for women doctors to admit that they encounter abuse. Overall, very few dentists (N=41) have admitted to experiencing violence, with physical violence at 7 per cent, verbal violence 49 per cent, and sexual violence 7 per cent. We must bear in mind that because dentists work in small and closed offices, with limited staff and in intimate proximity to patients, it may have been even more embarrassing for them to admit that they had faced violence, and therefore this may have contributed to under-reporting.

Nurses (N=199) revealed that they had faced much higher rates of all types of violence in comparison to doctors, with experiences of physical violence ranging from 46 to 54 per cent, verbal violence from 68 to 93 per cent, and sexual violence from 27 to 64 per cent. Similarly, LHWs (N=49) experienced high rates of violence, with physical violence ranging from 44 to 100 per cent, verbal violence from 71 to 100 per cent, and sexual violence from 33 to 68 per cent. Perhaps the anonymous nature of the survey encouraged some respondents to admit to experiencing violence but we have to be careful about generalizing these results as many women might still not have been entirely honest about their experience in order to protect the status of their profession. Chi-square significance results for degree and violence are highly significant, with physical violence ($X^2$= 69.020, p<.001), verbal violence ($X^2$= 58.863, p<.001), and sexual violence ($X^2$= 76.021, p<.001). The results indicate that although higher status degree holders encounter less of all types of violence, in comparison to nurses and LHWs, they face greater violence than doctors and dentists. The absolute results imply that regardless of the level of the degree held and consequent status, violence is a pervasive reality for all women healthcare practitioners.

Violence faced by women healthcare practitioners was correlated with their department, as set out in Table 4. There was greater sampling of departments where a greater number of women practitioners worked, largely due to the demands of segregation, including General Medicine, Critical Care, Surgery, Maternity, Emergency, and Paediatrics. Violence was found to prevail across all the 19 departments and Chi-square associations were found significant for physical violence ($X^2$= 88.269, p<.001), verbal violence ($X^2$= 85.720, p<.001), and sexual violence ($X^2$= 51.434, p<.05). Departments in which women healthcare practitioners suffered high rates of physical violence included the oncology ward (75 per cent), emergency (73 per cent), CCU (54 per cent), nephrology (50 per cent), and the maternal and obstetrics ward (50 per cent). Verbal violence was dominant in the cancer ward: chemotherapy (100 per cent), radiology (80 per cent), oncology (75 per cent), general medicine (85 per cent), maternal care and obstetrics (80 per cent), CCU (81 per cent), emergency (81 per cent), and the paediatric department (71 per cent). Sexual violence was found to be highly prevalent in the general medicine (55 per cent), chemotherapy (63 per cent), and the emergency ward (47 per cent). Most of these departments are highly stressful zones where the risk to patient mortality is high and thus violence against women practitioners is greater.

Women healthcare practitioners across different designations also faced considerable violence, as set out in Table 5. Chi-square results show that physical violence ($X^2$= 81.870, p<.001), verbal violence ($X^2$= 111.859, p<.001), and sexual violence ($X^2$= 55.851, p<.005) are highly significant realities for women practitioners across the designations that they hold. Doctors with higher designations encounter less of all types of violence, for example, junior house officers indicated suffering significant violence (physical violence at 14 per cent, verbal violence at 65 per cent, and sexual violence at 18 per cent), whereas senior consultants suffered none of these. However, assistant professors and postgraduate residents indicated suffering from violence and thus the limited sample results must be read and interpreted with caution. There was no significant difference in the level of seniority and experience of violence amongst nurses and LHWs. Although staff nurses are considerably junior to assistant superintendent nurses, the comparative level of violence directed towards them was shown to be 46 per cent as against 77 per cent respectively for physical violence, 90 per cent versus 94 per cent respectively for verbal violence, and 53 per cent versus 65 per cent respectively for sexual violence. Similarly, the senior designated LHS faced nearly the same rate of all three types of violence in comparison to the subordinate LHW. It appears that regardless of seniority and professional qualification, violence is faced by all women healthcare practitioners, especially nurses and LHWs.

### Table 3

Frequency and Chi-square results for violence experienced by women healthcare practitioners in Pakistan according to degree.

| | Total f (%) | Experienced PV f (%) | Experienced VV f (%) | Experienced SV f (%) |
|---|---|---|---|---|
| **Doctors** | | | | |
| Bachelor of Medicine, Bachelor of Surgery (MBBS) | 94 (23.4) | 16 (17.8) | 59 (65.6) | 16 (17.8) |
| Fellowship of the College of Physicians and Surgeons (FCPS) | 16 (04.0) | 06 (37.5) | 09 (56.3) | 06 (37.5) |
| MBBS with MPhil. and PhD in Public Health | 02 (00.5) | 01 (50.0) | 02 (100.0) | 01 (50.0) |
| | *112 (27.9)* | *23 (20.5)* | *70 (62.5)* | *23 (20.5)* |
| **Dentist** | | | | |
| Bachelor of Dental Surgery (BDS) | 36 (09.0) | 03 (08.3) | 16 (44.4) | 03 (08.3) |
| Master of Dental Surgery (MDS) | 04 (01.0) | – | 03 (75.0) | – |
| Restorative Dental Science (RDS) | 01 (00.2) | – | 01 (100.0) | – |
| | *41 (10.2)* | *03 (07.3)* | *20 (48.8)* | *03 (07.3)* |

|  | Total f (%) | Experi-enced PV f (%) | Experi-enced VV f (%) | Experi-enced SV f (%) |
|---|---|---|---|---|
| **Nurses** |  |  |  |  |
| BA/BSc Nursing | 105 (26.2) | 57 (54.3) | 96 (91.4) | 67 (63.8) |
| Diploma | 44 (11.0) | 21 (47.7) | 41 (93.2) | 12 (27.3) |
| Matric | 28 (07.0) | 14 (50.0) | 21 (75.0) | 14 (50.0) |
| MSc Nursing | 22 (05.5) | 10 (45.5) | 15 (68.2) | 11 (50.0) |
|  | *199 (49.6)* | *102 (51.2)* | *173 (77.4)* | *104 (52.3)* |
| **LHWs** |  |  |  |  |
| FSc Examination | 41 (10.2%) | 18 (43.9%) | 30 (73.2%) | 28 (68.2%) |
| Middle School (Grade 8) | 07 (01.7) | 04 (57.0) | 05 (71.4) | 02 (33.3) |
| Pharmacy Technician Course | 01 (00.2) | 01 (100.0) | 01 (100.0) | - |
|  | *49 (12.2)* | *23 (46.9)* | *36 (73.4)* | *30 (61.2)* |
| Chi-square Significance, p value |  | 69.020 <0.001 | 58.863 <0.001 | 76.021 <0.001 |
| **Total** | 401 (100%) | 151 (37.7%) | 299 (74.6%) | 160 (39.9%) |
| **Key**: PV: Physical Violence, VV: Verbal Violence, SV: Sexual Violence | | | | |

**Table 4**

Frequency and chi-square results for violence experienced by women healthcare practitioners in Pakistan according to department.

|  | Total f (%) | Experi-enced PV f (%) | Experi-enced VV f (%) | Experi-enced SV f (%) |
|---|---|---|---|---|
| **General Medicine** | 95 (23.7) | 24 (25.3) | 81 (85.2) | 52 (54.7) |
| **LHWs** | 49 (12.2) | 23 (46.9) | 36 (73.4) | 30 (61.2) |
| **Gynaecology** |  |  |  |  |
| Extended programme for immunization (EPI) | 5 (01.2) | 02 (40.0) | 03 (60.0) | 02 (40.0) |

|  | Total f (%) | Experienced PV f (%) | Experienced VV f (%) | Experienced SV f (%) |
|---|---|---|---|---|
| Maternal Care and Obstetrics | 55 (13.7) | 28 (50.9) | 44 (80.2) | 15 (27.3) |
| **Critical Care Unit (CCU)** | 37 (09.2) | 20 (54.1) | 30 (81.1) | 07 (18.9) |
| **Dental Department** |  |  |  |  |
| Orthodontics | 10 (02.5) | - | 05 (50.0) | - |
| Oral Surgery | 11 (02.7) | - | 05 (45.5) | - |
| Surgery | 20 (05.0) | 03 (15.0) | 10 (50.0) | 10 (50.0) |
| **Cancer Ward** |  |  |  |  |
| Oncology | 08 (02.0) | 06 (75.0) | 06 (75.0) | 02 (25.0) |
| Chemotherapy | 08 (02.0) | 02 (25.0) | 08 (100.0) | 05 (62.5) |
| Radiotherapy | 10 (06.5) | 05 (50.0) | 08 (80.0) | 05 (50.0) |
| **Nephrology Department** |  |  |  |  |
| Nephrology | 16 (04.0) | 08 (50.0) | 11 (68.8) | 03 (18.8) |
| Dialysis Unit | 6 (01.5) | 01 (16.7) | 02 (33.3) | 01 (16.7) |
| Urology | 2 (00.5) | 01 (50.0) | 02 (100.0) | - |
| **Emergency** | 15 (04.0) | 11 (73.3) | 12 (80.7) | 07 (46.7) |
| **Ophthalmology** | 12 (03.0) | 03 (25.0) | 07 (58.3) | 06 (50.0) |
| **Out-Patient Department (OPD)** | 8 (02.0) | 03 (37.5) | 04 (50.0) | 03 (37.5) |
| **Paediatric** | 14 (03.5) | 05 (33.3) | 10 (71.4) | 05 (33.3) |
| **ENT** | 3 (00.7) | - | 01 (100.0) | - |
| **Basic Science Demonstrators** |  |  |  |  |
| Physiology | 1 (00.2) | 01 (100.0) | 01 (100.0) | 01 (100.0) |
| Biochemistry | 2 (00.5) | 01 (50.0) | 01 (50.0) | 01 (50.0) |
| **Gastroenterology** | 3 (00.7) | 02 (66.7) | 03 (100.0) | - |
| **Healthcare Department** | 3 (00.7) | - | 03 (100.0) | 01 (33.3) |
| **X-Ray Department** | 2 (00.5) | - | 02 (100.0) | 01 (50.0) |

| | Total f (%) | Experi-enced PV f (%) | Experi-enced VV f (%) | Experi-enced SV f (%) |
|---|---|---|---|---|
| Dermatology | 2 (00.5) | 01 (50.0) | 02 (100.0) | 01 (50.0) |
| Neurosurgery | 2 (00.5) | 01 (50.0) | 01 (50.0) | 01 (50.0) |
| Orthopaedic | 1 (00.2) | - | 01 (100.0) | 01 (100.0) |
| Pharmacology | 1 (00.2) | - | - | - |
| Chi-square significance, p value | | 88.269 <0.001 | 85.720 <0.001 | 51.434 <0.05 |
| Total | 401 (100%) | 151 (37.7%) | 299 (74.6%) | 160 (39.9%) |
| Key: PV: Physical Violence, VV: Verbal Violence, SV: Sexual Violence | | | | |

### Table 5

Frequency and Chi-square results for violence experienced by women healthcare practitioners in Pakistan according to designation.

| | Total f (%) | Experi-enced PV f (%) | Experi-enced VV f (%) | Experi-enced SV f (%) |
|---|---|---|---|---|
| Doctors | | | | |
| Postgraduate Resident (PGR) | 16 (04.0) | 08 (50.0) | 11 (68.8) | 04 (18.2) |
| House Officer (HO) | 63 (15.7) | 09 (14.3) | 41 (65.1) | 11 (17.5) |
| Women Medical Officer (WMO) | 10 (02.5) | 01 (20.0) | 05 (50.0) | 03 (30.0) |
| Surgeon | 05 (01.2) | - | 02 (40.0) | 01 (20.0) |
| Senior Consultant | 01 (00.2) | - | - | - |
| Attaché-District Office Doctor | 09 (02.2) | 02 (22.2) | 05 (55.6) | 02 (22.2) |
| Resident Medical Officer | 03 (00.7) | 01 (33.3) | 02 (66.7) | - |
| Lecturer | 03 (00.7) | 02 (66.7) | 03 (100.0) | 01 (33.3) |
| Assistant Professor | 02 (00.5) | - | 01 (50.0) | 01 (50.0) |
| | 112 (27.9) | 23 (20.5) | 70 (62.5) | 23 (20.5) |

| | Total f (%) | Experienced PV f (%) | Experienced VV f (%) | Experienced SV f (%) |
|---|---|---|---|---|
| **Dentist** | | | | |
| Master of Dental Surgery (MDS)/FCPS Trainee | 16 (04.0) | 02 (12.5) | 08 (50.0) | 02 (12.5) |
| Dental Surgeon | 25 (06.2) | 01 (04.0) | 12 (48.0) | 01 (04.0) |
| | *41 (10.2)* | *03 (07.3)* | *20 (48.8)* | *03 (07.3)* |
| **Nurse** | | | | |
| Assistant Superintendent | 17 (04.2) | 13 (76.5) | 16 (94.1) | 11 (64.7) |
| Nurse Instructor | 13 (03.2) | 07 (53.8) | 10 (76.9) | 07 (53.8) |
| Staff Nurse | 107 (26.7) | 49 (45.8) | 96 (89.7) | 57 (53.3) |
| Superintendent Nurse | 02 (00.5) | 02 (100.0) | 02 (100.0) | - |
| Head Nurse | 49 (12.2) | 28 (57.1) | 39 (79.5) | 23 (46.9) |
| Trainee Nurse | 09 (02.2) | 02 (22.2) | 08 (88.9) | 06 (66.7) |
| Nurse Principal | 02 (00.5) | 01 (50.0) | 02 (100.0) | - |
| | *199 (49.6)* | *102 (51.2)* | *173 (77.4)* | *104 (52.3)* |
| **LHW** | | | | |
| Midwife LHW | 10 (02.5) | 03 (30.0) | 02 (20.0) | 06 (60.0) |
| LHS | 03 (00.7) | 01 (33.3) | 02 (66.7) | 03 (100.0) |
| LHW | 36 (09.0) | 19 (52.8) | 32 (88.9) | 21 (58.3) |
| | *49 (12.2)* | *23 (46.9)* | *36 (73.4)* | *30 (61.2)* |
| Chi-square Significance, p value | | 81.870 <0.001 | 111.859 <0.001 | 55.851 <0.005 |
| **Total** | 401 (100) | 151 (37.7) | 299 (74.6) | 160 (39.9) |

**Key:** PV: Physical Violence, VV: Verbal Violence, SV: Sexual Violence

## *Workplace violence across categories of perpetrators and responses of victims*

There are three principal types of perpetrators who inflict

violence on women healthcare practitioners, including patients, family attendants, and co-workers, as set out in Table 6. Verbal violence was the most frequent abuse against women practitioners, with family attendants being the most frequent perpetrators at 58 per cent and patients and co-workers following at 38 and 30 per cent respectively. With regard to physical violence, family attendants were labelled as the most common perpetrators at 26 per cent, with patients and co-workers following at 21 and 12 per cent respectively. The findings relating to sexual violence again indicated that family attendants are the most likely perpetrators at 33 per cent, with patients and co-workers following at 22 and 12 per cent, respectively. The findings make it evident that women practitioners pay a high price for the unregulated management of family attendants in Pakistan's public health sector. The absence of strict regulation in public sector hospitals in relation to timing and the number of family attendants accompanying each patient may be responsible. However, the cultural attitudes of family attendants, who view women practitioners as easy targets for their frustrations, also play a major role here.

The responses of women respondents during and after experiencing different types of violence were also studied (Table 7). Alarmingly, but not unexpectedly for this region, the most common response of victims was either to take no action at all (physical violence: 80 per cent, verbal violence: 88 per cent, sexual violence: 71 per cent) or to pretend that nothing exceptional had occurred (physical violence: 60 per cent, verbal violence: 63 per cent, sexual violence: 30 per cent). Some respondents did disclose that they told the perpetrators to stop and shared their victimization with colleagues and seniors. However, of alarm was that a negligible number of respondents attempted to enlist the assistance of unions (physical violence: 0.2 per cent, verbal violence: 3 per cent, sexual violence: 2 per cent), sought the services of other medical practitioners and counsellors (physical violence:1 per cent, verbal violence: 1 per cent, sexual violence: 0.2 per cent), or pursued prosecution (physical violence: 0.2 per cent, verbal violence: 0 per cent, sexual violence: 0.2 per cent). The findings reveal that women healthcare practitioners in Pakistan are contributing to the individual and wider social risks resulting from violence in terms of: (a) accepting violence passively and encouraging perpetrators, (b) not seeking medical attention and placing themselves at the risk of physical and psychological harm, and (c) not pursuing accountability to deter future victimization against themselves and other working women.

The emotional consequences suffered by women practitioners after experiencing violence are summarized in Table 8. A considerable number of women victims expressed moderate levels of suffering such as: (1) having repeated, disturbing memories, thoughts, or images of the attack (physical violence: 14 per cent, verbal violence: 27 per cent, sexual violence: 11per cent); (2) having to avoid thinking or speaking about the attack or having upsetting feelings relating to it (physical violence: 16 per cent, verbal violence: 28 per cent, sexual violence: 14 per cent); (3) becoming extremely cautious and on guard in their work environments (physical violence:14 per cent, verbal violence: 29 per cent, sexual violence: 11 per cent); and (4) having feelings that continuation of work has become an effort for them (physical violence:15 per cent, verbal violence: 25 per cent, sexual violence: 13 per cent).The findings suggest that women in the region have been well socialized into accepting violence and ill-equipped to recognize the enduring psychosomatic consequences of victimization. Only a few women felt they needed to take time off from work after facing violence. This may be because public sector hospitals deduct the salaries of employees who take leave from work and it is not easy for women victims to prove victimization and consequently obtain permission for official paid leave.

### Table 6

Frequency of violence imposed upon women healthcare practitioners in Pakistan according to the type of male perpetrator.

|  | Imposed PV $f$ (%) | Imposed VV $f$ (%) | Imposed SV $f$ (%) |
|---|---|---|---|
| Patient | 82 (20.5) | 172 (37.7) | 107 (21.6) |
| Family attendant | 104 (25.9) | 231 (57.6) | 133 (33.2) |
| Co-worker | 48 (12.0) | 117 (29.2) | 49 (12.2) |

### Table 7

Frequency of responses by women healthcare practitioners in Pakistan after experiencing violence.

|  | Experienced PV $f$ (%) | Experienced VV $f$ (%) | Experienced SV $f$ (%) |
|---|---|---|---|
| No action | 33 (80.2) | 72 (88.0) | 43 (70.7) |
| Tried to defend myself | 48 (12.0) | - | 50 (12.5) |
| Told the person to stop | 71 (17.7) | 152 (37.9) | 39 (09.7) |
| Told family and friends | 31 (7.7) | 45 (11.2) | 25 (06.2) |
| Told a colleague | 45 (11.2) | 108 (26.9) | 18 (04.5) |
| Transferred to another position | 09 (2.2) | 09 (2.2) | 05 (1.2) |
| Reported to senior staff member | 73 (18.2) | 132 (32.9) | 36 (09.0) |

|  | Experienced PV f (%) | Experienced VV f (%) | Experienced SV f (%) |
|---|---|---|---|
| Pretended it did not happen | 40 (59.9) | 93 (63.2) | 39 (29.7) |
| Sought help from union | 01 (0.2) | 11 (02.7) | 07 (1.7) |
| Sought medical attention/ counselling | 03 (0.7) | 05 (01.2) | 01 (0.2) |
| Pursued prosecution | 01 (0.2) |  | 01 (0.2) |

## Table 8

Frequency of consequences suffered by women healthcare practitioners in Pakistan after facing violence.

|  | Experienced PV f (%) | Experienced VV f (%) | Experienced SV f (%) |
|---|---|---|---|
| **Repeated, disturbing memories, thoughts, or images of the attack?** |  |  |  |
| Not at all | 63 (15.7) | 133 (33.2) | 11 (02.7) |
| Moderately | 55 (13.7) | 107 (26.7) | 42 (10.5) |
| Extremely | 26 (06.5) | 39 (9.7) | 59 (14.7) |
| **Avoided thinking or speaking about the attack/avoided nurturing feelings related to it?** |  |  |  |
| Not at all | 58 (14.5) | 127 (31.7) | 10 (02.5) |
| Moderately | 65 (16.2) | 111 (27.7) | 55 (13.7) |
| Extremely | 21 (05.2) | 39 (9.7) | 47 (11.7) |
| **Being extra-alert, watchful, and on guard?** |  |  |  |
| Not at all | 57 (14.2) | 125 (31.2) | 11 (2.7) |
| Moderately | 56 (14.0) | 115 (28.7) | 45 (11.2) |
| Extremely | 31 (07.7) | 38 (09.5) | 56 (14.0) |
| **Feeling that everything I did was an effort?** |  |  |  |
| Not at all | 59 (14.7) | 136 (33.9) | 14 (03.5) |
| Moderately | 61 (15.2) | 101 (25.2) | 51 (12.7) |
| Extremely | 24 (06.0) | 41 (10.2) | 48 (12.0) |

| | Experienced PV *f* (%) | Experienced VV *f* (%) | Experienced SV *f* (%) |
|---|---|---|---|
| **Have to take time off from work** | | | |
| No | 137 (34.2) | 263 (65.6) | 98 (24.4) |
| Yes | 17 (04.2) | 15 (03.7) | 14 (03.5) |
| **Length of leave** | | | |
| Hours | 08 (02.0) | 05 (1.2) | – |
| Days | 07 (01.7) | 13 (3.2) | 02 (0.5) |
| Weeks | 03 (00.7) | 02 (0.5) | 04 (1.0) |
| Months | 02 (00.5) | 06 (1.5) | 06 (1.5) |

## Workplace violence across odds of higher violence

Bivariate regression analysis is regularly used in public health and violence research to assess the odds of an event occurring. Statistics are set out in Table 9, using odds ratio (OR) and confidence intervals (CI). The regression results for this study show that younger women, between the ages of 20 and 39, are twice as likely to suffer all three types of violence (Odd ratio results: Physical Violence: OR 2.79, 95 per cent, CI 3.23–2.23; Verbal Violence: OR 3.78, 95 per cent, CI 4.68–2.26; and Sexual Violence: OR 2.72, 95 per cent, CI 1.58–4.69). Similarly, unmarried women without children also face higher odds of suffering from violence (Odd ratio results: Physical Violence: OR 1.47, 95 per cent, CI 1.06–2.07; Verbal Violence: OR 3.93, 95 per cent, CI 1.32–4.95; and Sexual Violence: OR 5.71, 95 per cent, CI 1.42–8.39). Unmarried women healthcare practitioners face an astonishing three times higher risk of verbal violence and a five times higher risk of sexual violence in comparison to married women healthcare providers. These results are not surprising as globally younger and unmarried women healthcare practitioners are known to face higher risk of violence (Neuman & Baron 1998). Not only are they more attractive victims, but their inexperience and lack of spousal guardianship make them easier targets for perpetrators.

Surprisingly, Muslim women face higher risk of all three types of violence in comparison to minorities such as Christians and Hindus, (Odd ratio results: Physical Violence: OR 1.65, 95 per cent, CI 1.00–2.72; Verbal Violence: OR 1.17, 95 per cent, CI 0.65–2.09; and Sexual Violence: OR 1.08, 95 per cent, CI 0.65–1.79). This may be because the public victimizes Muslim women healthcare practitioners for working in a man's field and feels it is justified in abusing them given their sullied existence, sealed by constant interaction with non-relative males. Alternatively, it may be that although Muslim women practitioners are in majority, the common expectation by the public is that most nurses are Christians or Hindus. This is because Muslim women are usually not permitted or encouraged to interact with non-relative males in the workforce. Therefore, it may be that the public practises greater violence against women practitioners who they falsely consider to be religious minorities with fewer opportunities to seek retribution.

Women healthcare practitioners with a lower income of below PKR 39,999 (Odd ratio results: Physical Violence: OR 1.71, 95 per cent, CI 1.07–1.33; Verbal Violence: OR 1.92, 95 per cent, CI 1.08–1.39; and Sexual Violence: OR 1.90, 95 per cent, CI 1.42–2.53); and on contractual employment (Odd ratio results: Physical Violence: OR 2.01, 95 per cent, CI 1.26–3.20; Verbal Violence: OR 1.58, 95 per cent, CI 1.08–2.54; and Sexual Violence: OR 1.86, 95 per cent, CI 1.06–1.63), are more vulnerable to all types of violence. Women workers with a lower socio-economic and professional status are known to face more of all types of violence, especially horizontal violence or professional bullying and sexual harassment. Again, perpetrators are encouraged by the knowledge that lack of privileged affiliations given their socio-professional inferiority will reduce the likelihood of women victims reporting or gaining justice against them in a patriarchal regime.

Nurses and LHWs face higher risk of all types of violence in comparison to doctors (Odd ratio results: Physical Violence: OR 2.36, 95 per cent, CI 1.78–3.12; Verbal Violence: OR 1.86, 95 per cent, CI 1.36–2.54; and Sexual Violence: OR 1.92, 95 per cent, CI 1.17–2.19). This is again an expected finding because nurses and LHWs are from a much lower social and occupational status. It is difficult for them to prevent violence against themselves or report it given fears of job loss and retribution, and this adds to the confidence of perpetrators. The following groups of women healthcare practitioners all face higher risk of violence:

(1) Work longer hours (Odd ratio results: Physical Violence: OR 1.69, 95 per cent, CI 1.09–2.62; Verbal Violence: OR 1.40, 95 per cent, CI 1.08–2.20; and Sexual Violence: OR 1.35, 95 per cent, CI 1.07–2.08).

(2) Work during night shifts (Odd ratio results: Physical Violence: OR 1.77, 95 per cent, CI 1.07–1.80; Verbal Violence: OR 2.27, 95 per cent, CI 1.34–3.84; and Sexual Violence: OR 1.45, 95 per cent, CI 1.06–2.21).

(3) Live in hospital provided accommodation (Odd ratio results: Physical Violence: OR 3.10, 95 per cent, CI 1.16–6.31; Verbal Violence: OR 4.09, 95 per cent, CI 1.89–6.84; and Sexual Violence: OR 1.29, 95 per cent, CI 1.05–2.85).

This is because night shifts and communal accommodation present greater dangers for women practitioners who are more easily found and followed by patients, attendants, and co-workers. Also, during night shifts, there is much less staff and security.

## Table 9

Bivariate regression results for women healthcare practitioners in Pakistan showing the odds of experiencing violence.

| | Odds of Higher PV OR (95% CI) | Odds of Higher VV OR (95% CI) | Odds of Higher SV OR (95% CI) |
|---|---|---|---|
| **Age in years** | | | |
| 20–29 | 2.79 (3.23–2.23)* | 3.78 (4.68–2.26)* | 2.72 (1.58–4.69)*** |
| 30–39 | 1.90 (0.82–2.45)* | 1.50 (0.78–2.23)* | 1.20 (0.87–2.56)*** |
| 40+ | 1 | 1 | 1 |
| **Marital Status** | | | |
| Never Married | 1.47 (1.06–2.07)** | 3.93 (1.32–4.95)* | 5.71 (1.42–8.39)** |
| Currently or once married (Widowed/divorced/separated) | 1 | 1 | 1 |
| **Religion** | | | |
| Islam | 1.65 (1.00–2.72)** | 1.17 (0.65–2.09) | 1.08 (0.65–1.79) |
| Minorities (Christian/Hindu) | 1 | 1 | 1 |
| **Children** | | | |
| None | 1.18 (0.77–1.81)* | 1.57 (0.93–2.13)* | 1.23 (0.75–2.01)* |
| Have children | 1 | 1 | 1 |
| **Income** | | | |
| ≤39,999 | 1.71 (1.07–1.33)* | 1.92 (1.08–1.39) | 1.90 (1.42–2.53)*** |
| ≥ 40,000 | 1 | 1 | 1 |
| **Residence** | | | |
| Hospital-provided | 3.10 (1.16–6.31)** | 4.09 (1.89–6.84)*** | 1.29 (1.05–2.85)* |
| Private | 1 | 1 | 1 |
| **Type of Women Healthcare provider** | | | |
| Nurse and LHW | 2.36 (1.78–3.12)*** | 1.86 (1.36–2.54)*** | 1.92 (1.17–2.19)* |
| Doctor | 1 | 1 | 1 |
| **Government contract** | | | |
| Contractual | 2.01 (1.26–3.20)*** | 1.58 (1.08–2.54)** | 1.86 (1.06–1.63)* |
| Permanent | 1 | 1 | 1 |
| **Government employee** | | | |
| Private or LHW | 1.79 (1.01–1.65)* | 1.70 (1.03–1.60)* | 1.54 (1.01–3.34)* |
| Government employee | 1 | 1 | 1 |
| **Works at private clinic in the evening** | | | |
| Yes | 1.65 (1.09–2.93)* | 1.22 (1.01–2.43) | 3.25 (1.78–5.93)*** |
| No | 1 | 1 | 1 |

|  | Odds of Higher PV OR (95% CI) | Odds of Higher VV OR (95% CI) | Odds of Higher SV OR (95% CI) |
|---|---|---|---|
| **Additional working hours after shift time** | | | |
| Yes | 1.69 (1.09–2.62)*** | 1.40 (1.08–2.20)* | 1.35 (1.07–2.08)* |
| No | 1 | | 1 |
| **Have to work night shifts** | | | |
| Yes | 1.77 (1.07–1.80)* | 2.27 (1.34–3.84)*** | 1.45 (1.06–2.21)** |
| No | 1 | 1 | 1 |

P-value significance: ***$p < 0.05$, **$p < 0.05$, *$p < 0.5$
Abbreviations: 1, reference category; OR, odds ratio; CI, confidence interval
Notes: Logistic regression analysis was carried out to obtain AOR after controlling for respondent illiteracy, low household income, and age (continuous variable)

# Conclusion

An attempt was made to collect empirical data from major regions of Pakistan in order to confirm the reality of workplace violence faced by women healthcare practitioners. Nearly all the respondents confirmed that they had suffered some form of violence in the past 12 months. Tests of association further clarified that regardless of employment, and organizational or socio-demographic characteristics, women suffered from verbal, physical, and sexual violence. Strong proof has been set out that violence is driven by socio-cultural beliefs. The male perpetrators of violence are listed as, at first rank, family attendants, at second rank, patients, and at third rank, co-workers. Verbal violence was the most frequent form of abuse suffered by women, followed by physical and sexual violence. Regression results reveal significant risk factors for higher odds of facing violence for women practitioners in Pakistan. As expected, younger and unmarried women face a greater risk of violence than older and married women. Women who work longer hours and have night shifts are also more vulnerable to facing abuse. Those earning lower salaries on contractual employment and living in hospital provided accommodation are also at a greater risk of violence. Finally, Muslim women overall, and nurses and LHWs in comparison to doctors suffer greater violence. There is little doubt that lower class and inferior professional status play a large role in encouraging perpetrators. The responses of the victims sadly corroborates the hypothesis that there is very little reporting of violence or attempt to gain punitive justice for women practitioners. Of the greatest alarm is that although victims suffer from serious emotional problems such as recurring memories of abuse and remaining perpetually on guard at the workplace, they did not seek medical help or union assistance.

# References

Aftab, Tahera (2007): *Inscribing South Asian Muslim Women: An Annotated Bibliogaphy & Research Guide* (Netherlands, Brill).

Akram, Muhammad, and Faheem Jehangir Khan (2007): 'Health care services and government spending in Pakistan', (Islamabad, Pakistan Institute of Development Economics).

Arif, Seema (2011): 'Broken wings: issues faced by female doctors in Pakistan regarding career development', *International Journal of Academic Research in Business and Social Sciences:* 1, 79.

Ayub, Romana, and Saad Siddiqui (2013): *Community Health Workers of Pakistan & Their Attrition* (North Carolina, USA, Lulu Press).

Azhar, Saira, et al. (2009): 'The role of pharmacists in developing countries: the current scenario in Pakistan', *Human Resources for Health,* 7 (1), 54.

Bahalkani, Habib Akhtar, et al. (2011): 'Job satisfaction in nurses working in tertiary level health care settings of Islamabad, Pakistan', *Journal of Ayub Medical College, Abbottabad:* 23, 130–3.

Bellot, Jennifer (2011): 'Defining and assessing organizational culture', *Nursing Forum* (46:Wiley Online Library): 29–37.

d'Oliveira, Ana Flávia Pires Lucas, et al. (2002): 'Violence against women in healthcare institutions: An emerging problem', *Lancet,* 359 (9318): 1681–5.

Giddens, Anthony (1979): *Central problems in social theory: Action, structure, and contradiction in social analysis,* (Berkeley, University of California Press).

Gulzar, Saleema A., et al. (2010): 'Promoting motivation towards community health care: A qualitative study from nurses in Pakistan', *Journal of Pakistan Medical Association,* 60 (6): 501.

Hashemi, Fatemeh, et. al. (2012): 'Factors associated with reporting nursing errors in Iran: A qualitative study', BMC Nursing, 11 (1): 20.

ILO/ICN/WHO/PSI (2003): International Labour Office (ILO), International Council of Nurses (ICN), World Health Organization (WHO), and Public Services International (PSI), 'Workplace Violence in the Health Sector- Questionnaire', <http://www.who.int/violence_injury_prevention/violence/interpersonal/en/WVquestionnaire.pdf>

Kamchuchat, Chalermrat, et al. (2008): 'Workplace violence directed at nursing staff at a general hospital in southern Thailand', *Journal of Occupational Health,* 50 (2): 201–7.

Kingston, Marilyn J., et al. (2004): 'Attitudes of doctors and nurses towards incident reporting: a qualitative analysis', *Medical Journal of Australia,* 181 (1): 36–9.

Lok, Peter, and John Crawford (1999): 'The relationship between commitment and organizational culture, subculture, leadership style and job satisfaction in organizational change and development', *Leadership and Organization Development Journal*, 20 (7): 365–74.

Neuman, Joel H., and Robert A. Baron (1998): 'Workplace violence and workplace aggression: Evidence concerning specific forms, potential causes, and preferred targets', *Journal of Management*, 24 (3), 391–419.

Nishtar, Sania (2006): 'The Gateway Paper: Health Systems in Pakistan: A Way Forward', Pakistan's Health Policy Forum, Islamabad, Pakistan.

Olsen, Wendy (2004): 'Triangulation in social research: qualitative and quantitative methods can really be mixed', *Developments in Sociology*, 20: 103–18.

Plowright, David (2011): *Using mixed methods: Frameworks for an integrated methodology* (California, United States, Sage Publications).

Rehman, Anis, et al. (2011): 'Pakistani medical students' specialty preference and the influencing factors', *JPMA, The Journal of the Pakistan Medical Association*, 61 (7): 713–18.

Saeed, Arzoo, and Hajra Ibrahim (2005): 'Reasons for the problems faced by patients in government hospitals: Results of a survey in a government hospital in Karachi, Pakistan', *Journal of Pakistan Medical Association*: (45): 55.

Watts, Charlotte, and Cathy Zimmerman (2002): 'Violence against women: Global scope and magnitude', *Lancet*, 359 (9313): 1232–37.

World Health Organization (2005): 'Health Statistics and Health Information Systems; 2008', *The Global Burden of Disease: 2004 update*.

Zafar, Naeem, and M. Norma Bustamante-Gavino, (2008): 'Breastfeeding and working full time experiences of nurse mothers in Karachi, Pakistan', *International Journal of Caring Sciences*, 1 (3): 132.

## NOTES

1. The three sampled cities include: (1) the capital of Pakistan, Islamabad, (2) the capital of Punjab, Lahore, and (3) the capital of Sindh, Karachi. Karachi and Lahore are also the two largest cities in Pakistan, each with a population of over 10 million people. The public sector hospitals in these cities are large. The frequency and ratios for inpatients and outpatients are therefore the highest in these three cities, with large rural and village populations also visiting these health centres given the availability of a wide range of specialist treatments.
2. Hospital sampling was done through a list of hospitals generated from the Pakistan Medical and Dental Council site.
3. BHU sampling was done through a list of centres generated from the Punjab Rural Support Programme website.

# 4

# Voiced Experiences of the Workplace: Learning by Listening

The principal objective of the qualitative phase of my research was to question women participants about the causes, precipitators, and risks at their workplaces which contributed to violence against them. My semi-structured interview guide was based on international scholarship, my own research experience, and feedback from pilot interviews which I had held with women practitioners when I was conceptualizing the research project. Over 56 per cent of the total population of Pakistan is based in the province of Punjab, which is where my interviews were conducted. Women healthcare practitioners from the rural and urban regions of Punjab were interviewed across a four year period, beginning from 2012. The qualitative interviews were a complex experience for me. Women participants unanimously agreed that violence was an inevitable reality for them. For instance, a nurse supervisor unequivocally stated, 'Women practitioners are beaten or abused daily in Pakistan.'

The unanimous appeal by women healthcare practitioners was that workplace violence be given urgent attention because it was more prevalent than its domestic counterpart. One of the reasons for this is the sheer numbers. Women have to deal with fewer men in their homes, whereas women healthcare practitioners have to interact daily with numerous men including co-workers, patients, and family attendants. More importantly, women within their homes may assume a subservient demeanour, fulfil their domestic roles to the satisfaction of men, and/or use the prayer mat as a buffer to prevent an onslaught of violence while women care-providers remain exposed given their job description of having to remain active and involved. Women expressed difficulty in being able to describe their experiences in vivid detail given their fear of reliving the brutal experience and fear of retribution by the perpetrators. Incidents were frequently reported in third person but subsequently when the women became more at ease, they admitted to having suffered similar violence themselves. It became evident that the women did want to discuss the high prevalence of violence but did not want to admit that they themselves had faced it, possibly due to long-standing habit of secrecy.

Many women wanted to share their experiences of violence but asked me not to include certain aspects of their stories in my final account because they feared that their stories might be traced back to them. I was caught in the dilemma of listening to narrations of victims who, given cultural restrictions, had not received counselling or sought medical recovery options. It became evident that while I could not help the individual women I interacted with, if through my work I was able to change to some degree policies and cultural attitudes, then that would be no mean contribution towards helping women practitioners in the long run. I did refer some participants to two clinical psychologists who had generously agreed to counsel victims in confidence and without a fee. However, to date, no participant has utilized the counselling services and that is probably because women in our society are trained to believe that therapy is a sign of mental weakness and that victimization is a norm not requiring any special medical attention.

Although I felt under immense pressure to vividly and honestly portray the women's narrations in order to make the fullest impact on policymakers and implementers, I had to decide to ensure complete anonymity that the women participants desired. In this context, I have refrained from citing the names of the participants, their region, the hospital setting, the medical college at which they worked, and designations. I have also narrated only partial experiences, as requested, and not the whole individual experiences of violence or the career histories to completely ensure anonymity. That is why the findings have been presented in thematic form and different women's voices have been quoted, where relevant, under each construct. The final presentation of the findings to identify the determinants of violence in this and the following two chapters thus preserves the promise I made to participants, that their stories or experiences would not and could not be traced back to them individually.

The best time to ask women healthcare practitioners at hospitals for interviews was the tricky period when they were off duty in the afternoon or evening, or when they arrived early for their shift. In the case of LHWs, I would wait at the BHU to see when I could request them for an interview, when they were at the unit, and not visiting homes in the community. With all women healthcare practitioners, what worked was to very casually introduce the topic for the interview and assure them that many others had previously spoken about the topic.[1] Women doctors were more difficult to interview in comparison to nurses and LHWs, possibly because they wanted to separate themselves from other women healthcare practitioners to retain their image of occupying a higher status.

Sometimes they did not wish to accept that violence against them was a norm but were eager to agree that it was extreme against nurses and LHWs.

Overall, women doctor participants agreed that women doctors in rural regions, those from poorer families, and those occupying lower positions in the hierarchy faced greater violence. This gave me an opening to ask them about what they had heard about violence faced by other women doctors. My task was not helped by the fact that there is an extreme shortage of nurses in public sector hospitals and therefore most of the time the ward heads were very reluctant to allow nurses to be distracted from their work for interviews. It was however much easier to discuss experiences of violence with nurses and LHWs than with women doctors.

The reality of public sector hospitals in Pakistan is a stark contrast to what is expected from a care centre. The hospitals are usually decrepit and unmaintained buildings with ramshackle furniture (beds and chairs), scattered across private rooms and wards. The linen and towels, even after dry-cleaning, do not look clean. The walls are gloss-washed with cheap paint and often with splattering of stains from catechu and betel leaf. Family attendants, including children and elders, from poor and rural areas are to be found deep in sleep sprawled in any available corridor space and outside the wards, ICUs, and the emergency departments. The gardens and entry areas outside the hospitals are also usually crammed with outpatients and family attendants, blocking not just the roads and entries to the hospital but also vital emergency driveways. Many women practitioners revealed that they were unable to engage in extended strikes for improved working conditions out of extreme sympathy for the thousands of the poor who were dependent upon them. It was this pity that the administration and the government exploited to undermine the possible gains from union mobilization and strikes.

The belief that BHUs are well-resourced and sophisticated clinical structures across communities is far from the truth. The LHWs I visited worked in derelict and resource-depleted units, with many interviews even taking place on floor mats given the lack of seating facilities. In many ways, BHUs are microcosms of large public sector hospitals. They are essentially ill-stocked and dilapidated little houses or rooms converted into health units. It is not uncommon to encounter donkey carts, mud or brick roads, and unhelpful male vendors while approaching BHUs. The locations which house these units are characteristically impoverished, conservative housing communities which are generally opposed to modern health solutions for the well-being of women and children.

It is assumed that working women will report violence against them to organizational and administrative heads or even to external accountability bodies such as the police because they are more knowledgeable and empowered than women victims sequestered within homes. I however found that all the working women I interviewed had faced some form of violence but never officially reported it. Thus, much of the material found through media reports, court records, and the literature review of existing scholarship set out in Chapter 1 of this book seem to be just the tip of the iceberg with regard to the actual prevalence and magnitude of workplace violence against women healthcare practitioners in Pakistan. During my visits to public sector hospitals in Pakistan, it was common not to find a medico-legal officer dealing with victims of sexual assault or other forms of abuse. If one was to be found, it was usually a male officer and no women representatives were part of the unit. Usually, when in search of officers dealing with victims of violence at the workplace, I was met with suspicious glances and asked to visit the forensics office.

In Pakistan, there are greater economic, social, and political inequalities faced by women and therefore the rates of gender-based violence within homes and at the organizational level are greater. Class and ethnic characteristics of both the perpetrator and the victim are key risk indicators for workplace violence. I found, as described in this and the following two chapters, that social distinction such as gender, wage, hierarchical position, ward-belonging, and remoteness of the hospital location can contribute to the risk of workplace violence. Aggravatingly, women healthcare practitioners in Pakistan face a combination of gender, class, and ethnic workplace harassment.[2] Women from remote and minority ethnicities with a lower social status are afforded fewer opportunities for growth at the workplace and also face greater violence. It is evident from a conflict-oriented and Marxist-feminist perspective that women healthcare practitioners are facing violence due to societal power imbalances. Violence is taking on dual motives in terms of suppressing women practitioners in order to maintain both eco-social and political hegemony. Culturally, workplace violence becomes a means of discouraging entry into the workplace and also to warn women employees that their bargaining power will always be weak.

## Culture and Patriarchy

### The girl-child and patriarchy

Being subjected to violence becomes inevitable at the very birth of a girl-child. In patriarchal societies such as Pakistan, the male-child is given a higher status and preferential treatment because he is considered to be of greater social and economic utility. A family with a larger number of sons is the recipient of greater social status and prestige, and a family with only daughters is pitied and shamed. The socio-economic liability of being a woman has licensed resentful fathers and brothers who abuse and victimize the girl-child within the house and also deprive them of basic human rights such as nutrition, education, and healthcare. Early socialization of men in their homes teaches them that they can get away with perpetration of violence against their mothers and sisters. After marriage, wives and daughter-in-laws are not treated any better. The cultural norm is to value them for their reproductive and domestic services, and to use oppression and violence against them to ensure they meet social expectations. Women who cannot bear children and have only borne female children are known to suffer the most through violent social tools such as shaming and neglect, divorce and denial of separation rights, physical abuse, and even homicide. The 'cycle of violence' continues against women at the workplace. Male relatives at home are so deeply socialized in violent behaviour against the women in the household that they replicate these behavioural patterns both in public and at work. A senior doctor explained how experiencing violence was a norm for both working and non-working women in the region:

Men [colleagues, patients, and family attendants] treat us [women healthcare practitioners] in the same way that they treat their women at home. It is normal for them to treat all women aggressively and with disrespect. For them we are not professionals, but first and foremost we are the women of this society that is why they abuse and harm us without remorse or second thought. It is what they have been taught in their homes.

A nurse described the importance of the role of child socialization in the manifestation of violence against women:

All men in our society are taught to be violent to women. The only way violence against women will end is by training [the male child] within the homes and in the community. Men need to treat their female relatives better and teach their sons to respect women. Only then will they treat women in the public and at work organizations better.

## Male ideologies and the culture of violence

The perpetration of violence against women practitioners is accepted as a cultural norm in Pakistani society which is socially condoned and religiously justified. The cultural forces that dictate such practices are rooted not just in present-day customs but in the historical and religious legacies of the region. Hindu, Buddhist, Islamic, and colonialist traditions have combined to sustain and perpetuate violence against women, rationalizing the act, and putting the onus on the victims. Women discussed how the feudal norms of tribal areas and villages also prevail in the urban areas of Pakistan. Men from feudal backgrounds not only commodify women as symbols of honour but are frequently abusive in relation to them as a badge of their manliness in conformity with and preservation of feudal traditions. For this their actions are regarded as praiseworthy and they are rarely held accountable for it. These cultural attitudes of men make them incapable of recognizing and respecting women practitioners for their skill and ability. A nurse explained how women practitioners must be prepared to enter into a profession that does not afford protection or support:

> If women want to become doctors, nurses, or LHWs in Pakistan, they have to be prepared to face multiple forms of discrimination and violence as this is the culture in our country. You must remember that the men have a strong network; they are all connected and supportive of one another on the basis of cultural ties. The hospital organizational culture, like the wider social culture, also accepts violence against us [women healthcare practitioners].

A doctor aptly described the influence of feudalism on work cultures and the treatment of working women:

> Our society is dominated by feudal culture. Even educated men are not civilized. Much of the male public has little knowledge about the work ethics of a hospital organization; they cannot understand how we [women practitioners] struggle to remain professional, fulfil our responsibilities, and meet time frames. They consider hospitals to be male territories where women practitioners are not recognized as legitimate professionals. It is unthinkable and unacceptable for them to accept directions or orders from us [women practitioners]. This is why we face so much violence from them, including abusive language, physical violence, and sexual harassment.

## Polygamy and sexual aggression

Although polygamous rights in Islam are accompanied and constrained by riders such as the necessity of permission from the first wife and strict regulations such as equal treatment of all wives, the practice has been grossly exploited. Secret second marriages or affairs that do not convert into marriage are quite common amongst medical professionals. Male practitioners are known to employ promiscuous banter, make false promises, and be sexually aggressive with women practitioners. The health setting is considered a matchmaking site, with religious and cultural rights manipulated by men in quest of prospective wives or fiancés. Participants discussed how women nurses and doctors from rural and disadvantaged backgrounds are highly susceptible to flirtations and advances from dissolute doctors under false pretexts. In the event of a woman practitioner succumbing and getting involved in an affair or a second marriage, her (and her children's) future, in terms of emotional stability, social status, and financial security are seriously compromised. A nurse described a specific experience of sexual harassment and the common occurrence of women getting trapped in affairs or second marriages:

> Three married male resident doctors made trouble for me and another nurse on night duty once. They had brought nihari[3] for dinner and asked us to join them. We were alone in the ward and had heard of instances of attempted rape in the hospital at night. We were scared. I heard one of the doctors, who had a newly born baby daughter call another male colleague from his cell phone and say 'Choochi bohat fit hai, a ja bohat maza ayega' ('The girls are really hot; come over and we'll have

some fun'). We declined politely saying that we had work to do, as we couldn't afford to antagonize these men. What is the best that they can offer us? A temporary affair or perhaps a second marriage? Some nurses and young doctors, and even some women patients get trapped by these married doctors. In fact, there are occasions when nurses and young doctors get trapped by male patients. For the men in our society all this is normal but the woman's life is ruined.

## Gender segregation as a cultural norm

Segregation across social institutions such as the family, education, and the workplace can promote among men an unhealthy approach to women. Although Pakistani society has succeeded in maintaining segregation in most formal structures, it has not been possible to eliminate the mixing of genders in the health sector. Primary and secondary schooling remains segregated across most of Pakistan with the result that men are unable to deal with non-segregation as medical students and young doctors. After segregated schooling, men face a culture shock when their conservative ideals are violated through constant exposure to women at the workplace. Their resultant frustrations and confusion are vented through the perpetration of different types of violence against women. It was also mentioned that men feel that women healthcare practitioners, who are choosing to study and work in a non-segregated environment, are providing them with an open invitation for advances and aggression.

The media was listed as a contributing factor to greater complexities relating to segregation and non-segregation. Social networking sites and cinema from the West and from

India depict men and women in modern relationships and in close interaction, as friends or lovers. Because men in Pakistan are unable to emulate norms from media socialization, they begin to deal with non-relative females at the workplace in a manner that can be offensive for women. The physical proximity of working in a hospital setting becomes a gateway for frustrated men, who are not accustomed to a non-segregated work environment and are not held accountable for their inappropriate behaviour with women. Incidents were reported of male doctors touching women healthcare practitioners during outpatient day (OPD) and clinical examinations. Even senior male doctors were witnessed to unnecessarily touch both female colleagues and female patients' private parts during examinations. A nurse described the clash between the informal and rigid social rules of segregation at the workplace and the frustrations of men working in a non-segregated setup:

Men and women in our society are not supposed to directly talk to each other. But men and women at the hospital settings have to talk, interact, and deal with each other. It is uncomfortable and unpleasant for both genders. During my viva, my PG (post-graduate) in-charge, a resident trainee doctor, was taking photographs of me. I felt uncomfortable at the time but didn't say anything because it was embarrassing and I couldn't ask him to stop doing so in front of the professor while my viva was in progress. A year and a half later, during my house job, he told me that he had saved his photographs of me and looked at them daily. I asked him why he had taken them without my permission. He replied, 'I thought you knew and wanted them taken.' Men in our society behave in such a manner because they are not able to handle studying and working with women. Touching us unnecessarily and taking pictures of us excites them.

A doctor explained how the influence of the media and globalization has made the men in the region incapable of coping with the disjunction with contemporary reality and the traditional norms of segregation:

I think the men are frustrated because they watch Western and Indian movies. Men who seem the most conservative about maintaining segregation at the hospital are usually those putting on an act and are most eager for night duties. This is because night duty gives them an opportunity to mix with women more freely as they have seen abroad and in movies. There are a lot of frustrated men who pretend to uphold segregation publically but behave differently when the crowd dissipates.

Another experienced doctor described how the specific responsibilities and roles of practitioners at the hospital setting were not conducive to maintaining segregation and yet, at the same time, provides frustrated male practitioners with an opportunity to become sexually aggressive:

Male and female doctors share the same offices, washrooms, and scrubbing areas in the hospital. This is a huge problem in a society where segregation is the norm. Male co-workers who normally never talk to us directly or make eye contact end up touching and groping us whenever they get an opportunity. Complete segregation is impossible in the hospital … and so is the complete eradication of violence against women healthcare practitioners.

## Low professional status

Most of the women healthcare practitioners who participated in the interviews said that the nursing and LHW professions have an extraordinarily low status in Pakistani society. Participants described being likened to 'maids' and 'cleaners' rather than professional practitioners. Cultural norms dictate that men believe that women who work outside the home are 'indecent' and 'ambitious'. It is normal to find men speaking to one other about how women healthcare practitioners choose to intermingle with male non-relatives given their frustrations as married women or their desire to have an affair as single women. In the event of harassment or abuse, it was common to hear men say about women healthcare practitioner victims that: 'they had asked for it' or 'they know to expect this'. Women participants said that they were not looked up to and respected as professionals, as were their counterparts in the West, but rather were regarded as being inferior and immoral and this is why many Pakistani women practitioners were eager to obtain employment abroad. The critical negligence of maternal benefits such as extended maternal leave, nursing rooms, and flexible working hours were pointed out. Working women are penalized and shamed by the community for leaving their newly-born babies at home and returning to work and this is reinforced by structural policies which neglect working mothers. It was unthinkable for both conservative middle-class and élite families to permit their daughters to become nurses. A nurse superintendent concluded that only a complete transformation of nurse identity would have the effect of mitigating violence against nurses:

Until rich and middle class families in Pakistan dream of
their daughters becoming nurses, the way they do for them to
become doctors, this profession will suffer and women nurses
will face repeated violence.

Another nurse lamented community perceptions of nurses:

Nursing is not considered a very important profession in
Pakistan... it is indeed considered a dirty profession! Many
family members asked me, 'Why do you want to lose your
respect by becoming a nurse?' But I did not have any other
choice. There are only two professions for women from middle
and lower class families in our country: teaching and nursing.
Everyone considers nurses to be untrained and uneducated
underlings of doctors who are fit only to clean up and follow
doctor's orders. People do not know that we study the same
books as doctors and that we have even more knowledge of
what is good for the patient [in comparison to doctors]. For
us to be able to help the public, we need to be given respect.

## Negative identity of practitioners providing maternal and child health services

Women practitioners who provide maternal and child health
services are regarded with great suspicion in Pakistan. Women
practitioners providing services for family planning, abortion,
and immunization, especially nurses and LHWs, are perceived
negatively and treated with abuse.

The Lady Health Programme of Pakistan has low
budgets, with LHWs getting paid very low salaries and some
participants revealing that they had not been paid their salaries

by the government for the past three months. Along with inadequate compensation, LHWs have to work in public zones and unfamiliar home spaces which are known to be dangerous and conflict-ridden areas for working women. Many women field workers, such as LHWs, home nurses, paramedical staff, and physiotherapists suffer from indirect victimization by becoming secondary targets of domestic violence or street violence.[4] It is not unusual to come across men in the community who handle loaded weapons and firearms, causing great uncertainty and fear. Besides these spatial and regional problems, the gravest problem of all is the non-acceptance by the community of 'sinful' LHWs. The public resents and rejects LHW intrusion in what are considered private family decisions relating to child-bearing, place of delivery, and choice of abortion and immunization.

The services of LHWs are rarely recognized as welfare initiatives for women and children but are rather labelled as Western conspiracies to prevent the birth of Muslim children and alter the submissiveness of Muslim women. A majority of such women practitioners are shamed and stigmatized by society for providing illegitimate and immoral services that go against the fabric of Pakistani society and (socially defined) Islamic laws. Their negative social standing is a critical concern for the safety of LHWs in Pakistan, who are likened to prostitutes selling illegal services for the destruction of the traditional social order. Community men have been known to regularly threaten LHWs and members of their families. Of further concern is the fact that LHWs work in their own neighbourhoods and their home addresses are public knowledge. They are commonly threatened at their doorstep or during their work rounds with death and assault if they continue their 'immoral' practices. Many unfortunately have succumbed to horrific episodes of brutal beatings, rape, and even homicide. An LHW described how her profession faced complete rejection and disgrace by community members on public and media platforms:

> It is very difficult to visit houses and do our jobs in the community. We have neither respect nor social standing. We are likened to prostitutes. They have even described us [LHWs] on FM radio as immoral women who visit houses with condoms to find willing clients.

An experienced nurse described how they were prevented from delivering services and having a beneficial impact on the health of women and children:

> Family attendants ensure that we [women nurses and doctors] do not talk to patients [mothers with newborn children] about healthy pregnancy gaps and nutritional needs. Even more unfortunate is that the immunization charts distributed by us are not taken seriously and most families do not allow their newborns to be immunized. We are regularly abused, dismissed, and disrespected by family attendants so that young mothers do not get an opportunity to listen to us.

An LHW described the difficulties and violence that they faced in delivering services given the community belief that they are dishonest and dishonourable workers:

> It is not enough that we are underpaid and that many of us have not been paid our salaries [PKR 14,000 per month] for the last three months ... but what is really depressing is that our hard-earned income is labelled as haram[5] by the community.

Even elderly women in the community do not take our advice if we recommend multivitamins or iodine salt for them. They think we work to harm them. We have been molested, shot at, and raped. It is a great sacrifice [that] we make for this community as LHWs. No amount of money can compensate us for what we suffer.

## Public misconception that most women nurses are Christian or tainted Muslims

Another contributory reason for high rates of violence against women nurses is that most of the wider public perceive them to be 'Christians' in Pakistan. This is because it is assumed that Muslim families would never allow their daughters to become nurse care-providers who talk to, deal with, and almost unthinkably have to 'touch', 'wash', or 'clean' men who were not their *mahram*s or immediate blood relatives. A majority of the men were more likely to resort to verbal harassment, sexual overtures, and unnecessary physical contact because they felt that Christian nurses were more receptive to 'loose' and 'licentious' behaviour. Besides, it was perceived that the religion and family background of Christian women practitioners permitted them greater 'freedom' and 'liberty'. This did not exempt Muslim nurses, known or recognized to be Muslims, from violence. In fact, Muslim nurses were considered to be 'tainted' and 'sinful' for their constant interaction and physical contact with non-relative males, and consequently they were victimized for their choice of profession. Overall, the general public targeted workplace violence against both Christian and Muslim women nurses through burdensome negative labels. A nurse described how social perceptions prevalent in the community had concluded that services delivered by nurses would only be performed by Christian women:

> The mindset and attitude is that only Christians would touch and clean the body parts of male non-relatives. Moreover, it is assumed that Christian nurses would more easily allow casual touching and inappropriate language in the course of their work. The Muslim women nurses and doctors also face violence because the men in the community think they should be punished for interacting with male non-relatives and co-workers. It is unthinkable that a Muslim woman would not be in her father's or husband's home after dusk. Women nurses and doctors on night duty are considered to have no morals and their families are considered not to have honour ... thus men feel justified in directing violence against them.

## Class-based violence against lower class women doctors

The combination of gender and class as a precursor to violence was highlighted. Women doctors from rural areas and from lower socio-economic backgrounds faced common bullying, horizontal violence, and even serious impact violence. Given the absence of structural protection in Pakistan, it is the strength of influential and wealthy families which protects women from professional discrimination and violence. Therefore, in Pakistan, only women doctors from higher socio-economic backgrounds remain immune to abuse. Women doctors from the upper class are easily discernible given their strong family connections and kinship ties, élite language codes, superior attire, and confident behaviour, all of which combine to create a curtain of protection for them against high impact violence. However, even upper class women doctors admitted that they had to endure low impact types of violence such as verbal violence, sexual harassment, and professional bullying. Many agreed that these forms of violence were accepted by women doctors as part of the professional package in a male-dominated occupation. A doctor described the link between class belonging and the perpetration of violence against women doctors:

> A doctor's coat can only save a woman from violence if she is being publicly chaperoned in a private car or if she is from a well-renowned and well-connected family of doctors.

Another female doctor described how even women doctors from the upper classes suffered from low impact violence:

> I and my colleagues from similar backgrounds face less severe forms of violence. However, women doctors from a low income background, remote districts (selected in government medical colleges by merit), and who live in hospital accommodation face greater harassment and violence. They are easily distinguished by male colleagues because they remain highly segregated in their own social groups and do not mix with high profile and second-generation doctors. However, do not imagine that women doctors from upper classes are completely immune from violence. We face a lot of bullying behaviour and even sexual harassment: men use humiliating and indecent language when we pass by. I can remember incidents from medical college such as boys tying our *dupattas*[6] to our seats during classes, fondling us as they passed by, and telling lies

about how some girls are secretly their girlfriends. There was a girl who was very tall and she was mercilessly bullied and called 'Tango'. I still have no idea what this term meant, I think it had something to do with her long legs, but she dropped out of medical college because she could not handle the shame of being bullied and verbally harassed.

## Reporting shame

Women described the existence of huge professional barriers against reporting of violence in the healthcare sector. Incidents of women reporting violence and then subsequently facing negative consequences which damaged their respect and career were narrated. Supervisors and colleagues unwilling to help and support victims were described as bystander perpetrators of violence. Besides, the reporting of violence by women practitioners leads to problems of secondary victimization through which seniors, colleagues, and even families resort to victim-blaming. The insensitive and accusatory attitudes of significant others in the lives of women practitioners not only results in mental trauma but also the decision to permanently absorb experiences of victimization. Women practitioners who report on violence became objects of bullying, further harassment, and stigmatization. They are removed from their wards and familiar surroundings through the strong male networks. In addition, there are numerous and compounding fears preventing violence being reported by women practitioners influenced by the hidden curriculum. Both the education system and clinical training informally and tacitly ingrains into woman practitioners profound fears regarding disclosure, such as having to suffer greater violence, professional retribution and job loss, and also inviting shame upon their family and children.

Special mention was made by women about their daughters and how by reporting experiences of violence, they would be passing on the shame to them and jeopardizing their position in society, and also the detrimental effect it would have when arranging marriages for them in the future. Women had been warned both by past experiences of colleagues and superiors that reporting violence would only invite disgrace and dishonour upon them at the workplace. With placements in government jobs and representation in unions also controlled by male members of the society, women also suffered in terms of discrimination and exclusion if they reported male-perpetrated violence. Tales of the ostracization of women victims who reported victimization were shared, such as being removed from work teams and not getting permission from other departmental heads for transfer into new wards. This made women victims unable to continue to work in the hospital setting and indirectly forced resignations and even abandonment of the profession. The lack of family and in-law support not only deterred women practitioners from reporting violence but also led to continual stress, leading to further vulnerability for victimization. A senior nurse summarized the reasons for non-reporting of violence:

> The thing is that in our society, we cannot tell off perpetrators, we cannot tell their relatives or ours, and we cannot report to the police. Men know this and that is why women are vulnerable to such behaviour and harassment. Sometimes we manage to go on one or two hour strikes. People in the hospital and media find out about it but then because of the fear of pay cuts, the appeals of family attendants, and the Medical

Superintendent, and due to risks of patient mortality, we go back to work. For us, family responsibilities (getting our monthly salary to cover costs at home) and professional ethics take precedence over our safety and respect. Does society thank us for this? No!

An LHW elaborated on the reasons relating to the family and household finances which deterred women practitioners from reporting violence:

If we go home and tell our family and in-laws that we face different forms of violence, we will lose all respect. Women victims are usually reprimanded for placing themselves in vulnerable positions by choosing to work outside the home. We are told to protect ourselves or change our behaviour in so as to deter perpetrators, implying indirectly that we are to blame! We live in a very sick-minded community where women can be accused of anything at all. As the money we earn is required to run the household, we cannot leave our job. Our family also does not want to lose the income we bring home. In such circumstances, we are under a lot of stress: we cannot share our experiences with anyone and neither can we seek justice from the law. In the end, avoiding regular harassment is a game we learn to master.

# Governance and Structure

## *Resource and staff shortages*

The public healthcare services are known for their shortage of resources: medicines, equipment, staffing, and overall budget allocations. Women healthcare practitioners described the deplorable dual evils of corruption and violence in and by the health administration and senior male practitioners. Frustrations of practitioners, patients, and family attendants are a pulsating reality, as mortality rates and recovery times are constantly affected by resource failures. Women participants described how the public is aggressive and the relationship between employees is perpetually strained due to the grave shortages in staffing and resources. Women practitioners face the brunt of maltreatment stemming from health service inefficiencies. As violence against women practitioners has remained unchallenged in the region, even relatively passive male members of society have begun demonstrating explosive rage against women practitioners in the face of resource constraints. Senior doctors commonly vent their anger on junior women healthcare practitioners, especially when there are medical and procedural errors due to shortages and blame needs to be shifted to a subordinate. Women practitioners are usually easy targets for violence at the hands of men given their weaker physique and consequent inability to fight back, whereas perpetrators are unwilling to vent their aggression on male practitioners given the higher risk of immediate retribution.

There is also the critical issue of inadequate provision to poor patients in public sector health resources. Senior male doctors who own private practices, clinics, and hospitals were described as not coming for their rounds for many days. There is limited accountability of senior male practitioner performance and attendance by the male-dominated administration, with male colleagues (such as principals and junior doctors) supporting this form of corruption to develop their own networks of private practice. A senior nurse ward-head described in detail the realities of working in a public sector hospital and the distress caused to practitioners by shortages:

> Patients expect government hospitals to be like expensive private hospitals. Let me tell you what resources and staffing issues we have to deal with—only two nurses are allocated to a ward with 60 to 70 patients at a time. Each patient has a number of family attendants, who we have to deal with as well ... it is not just the 70 patients! There are a horde of people to judge, criticize, and abuse us on every bed. Nurses are beaten or abused by male patients, family attendants, and doctors on a daily and hourly basis.

A nurse described the high dependence on adequate resources and staffing for care outcomes and patient safety:

> Health outcomes do not just depend on our tireless efforts but on the availability of adequate staff, operational equipment, and life-saving medicines. Even though we undertake intensive scrubbing and theatre work for over 8 hours a day, we cannot compensate for the shortages in staffing and resources. I cannot describe the stress we face. When patients and family attendants find that treatment delays, long recovery times, and mortality are caused by shortages, they vent their frustration and anger on us [women nurses].

A doctor working in the general medicine ward described how male co-workers, and especially seniors, take out their work stress on women colleagues:

> Although violence against women is an accepted phenomenon

in our society, the long hours of work and shortage of staff and resources does not help matters. Shortages cause delays in treatment and errors in the hospital and male practitioners are not the kind to accept blame from patients and family attendants. Instead, they blame us [women practitioners]. We suffer from verbal and physical assault and are also usually blamed for errors because women are always easy targets for outbursts of frustration and blame.

## Professional bullying

In the public sector hospital organization of Pakistan, as in other work organizations here, there is an inability to discern between workplace bullying and the legitimate exercise of managerial authority. This is because women first receive early socialization within their homes regarding the acceptance of undeserved bullying from parents, elders, and male relatives, and second because of an absence of guidance in the educational curriculum and ongoing training about what constitutes workplace rights. At the secondary stage of socialization, the hidden curriculum of the health sector teaches women to remain submissive and passively accept professional bullying and workplace violence. Women practitioners face professional bullying at the hands of a range of co-worker bullies, including: (1) medical school and clinical instructor bullies, (2) imitating male co-worker bullies, (3) principal, the administration, and heads of department gatekeepers (who negotiate the sustenance of violence against women practitioners), and (4) supervisory two-headed snakes (who covertly condone violence against victims). The problem with bullying is that while it may at times be overt, it is often covert and unidentifiable. Indeed, structural policies such as restricting women's participation in hospital administration and governance are not considered to be horizontal violence but rather as a community service because they enable women to shoulder less of a professional burden and to fulfil their household responsibilities.

Women feel humiliated and degraded by male superiors and colleagues who do not respect their professional judgments or treat them as equal partners in the healthcare team. Some senior doctors were viewed as typical hysterical individuals who shamed women practitioners, especially nurses, in emergency settings and surgical wards to cover up their own shortcomings and errors. Direct supervisors, such as nurse supervisors, male professors, departmental heads, and clinical instructors, were described as constant critics who falsely accused and undermined women practitioners behind closed doors and contributed to low women practitioner identity at the workplace, especially in the presence of patients and family attendants. Given this onslaught from different categories of bullies, women practitioners were socialized to remain submissive and to assume subservient positions, thus contributing to the permanence of glass ceilings. The prevailing horizontal violence of male colleagues has a twofold impact: first, patients and family attendants emulate superior male doctors in disrespecting women practitioners, and second, it encourages the limited number of women supervisors to also become bullies in order to retain their positions. In the final analysis, professional bullying has prevented women from gaining opportunities for advancement and participation in governance. A doctor described the culture of relations between the instructors and trainees in the health sector:

Our instructors and demonstrators from medical school bully and exploit us: we are not encouraged to learn or raise queries. We are taught to sweep problems and gaps in knowledge under the carpet. Women medical and nursing students learn to remain silent and passive, or else face the consequences of discrimination and harassment. The administration and senior doctors with influence are all male and they keep us voiceless ... we have few opportunities to change the status quo. We must accept their mistreatment and their misdemeanours or else face more bullying and harassment.

A nurse shed light on the disloyalty of women supervisors in a male dominated work sector:

Our [women practitioners'] progress is inadequate in terms of on-the-job training and promotions in comparison to that of our male colleagues. Nurse supervisors and some heads of department [doctors], for example like in the gynaecology wards, are women but they are not supportive or united in matters related to women practitioner status, safety, and autonomy. To retain their position and get more benefits, they are in league with male administrations and contribute to keeping women practitioners oppressed in the hospital setting.

An experienced doctor added how abusive co-workers set a bad precedent for patients and family attendants in the accepted organizational treatment of women practitioners:

We [women practitioners] face a lot of bullying and abuse from male doctors because they consider themselves superior to us; after all, they live in bigger houses, drive expensive cars, and get paid much more than us. They don't realize that the hospital would not be able to function without us; it would simply have to close down! It is because doctors and senior administrators are rude and disrespectful to us that patient and family attendants also abuse us.

## VIP culture

Pakistani society is known for its VIP culture which comprises strong male networks of rich feudal families, businessmen, bureaucrats, and politicians. Hospital administrations in the public sector reserve special resources, staff, and rooms for the Pakistani élite. Besides, VIPs are given a special allowance and protection during their stay or visit to the hospital. Kinship and professional networks encourage men to practice the traditions of violence with ease, as women practitioners are without male relatives and administrative security in the clinical setting. The strong ties between the élites and the hospital administrations present a strong bulwark against the reporting of victimization faced by women. Women victims are socialized to remain 'calm' and 'dignified' during assault. A staff nurse described a specific incident of sexual harassment that she suffered at the workplace and the response of her senior colleagues in helping her to seek accountability from the perpetrator:

> I was visiting a private room on the third floor of the hospital reserved for bureaucrats and politicians. A middle-aged family attendant opened the door and pulled me inside roughly. I turned around to escape, shouting, 'Let go of me'. He grabbed my dupatta from behind and pulled again just as I was leaving the room. My head-scarf remained pinned on but my dupatta

had been ripped off. I left it behind and ran out. I went straight
to my department head, a senior professor. I was shaking and
furious but also very scared. I probably would not have reported
the incident but I wanted my dupatta back. How could I go
home without it; what would my family say? Professor saab[7]
made me sit in his office and after 20 minutes or so, the MS
[medical superintendent] came into the room followed by
the perpetrator. He started calling me 'Beti' [daughter] and
kept repeating that there had been a misunderstanding. My
professor was completely silent and did not rebuke the rich
man. When I began swearing on my parents' lives that he had
assaulted me, my professor quickly thanked the VIP and asked
him to go back and check on his patient, and leave him to
handle matters here. Then my professor explained to me: 'I
apologize on behalf of men like this but many nurses face such
problems. This commonly happens in the hospital. You are very
sensitive. You must stay calm and handle such incidents better
and try not to upset the entire hospital.'

## Verbal harassment

There is a specific language of harassment used against women
healthcare practitioners in Pakistani society which aims to
demean, humiliate, and shame them. Lower impact verbal
violence such as bullying, defamation, or swearing is made to
appear to be a minor offence inflicting no real damage to the
victim. In this way, the healthcare systems and processes of
accountability are not geared towards mitigating or shaming
verbal violence. Two types of language codes are used by men
in the hospital setting: one that is overtly abusive and another
that is covertly offensive. The second form of expression took

time to get used to involving as it did double entendre and sexual puns. Younger women practitioners who are not well-versed in the threats they face are more vulnerable targets for violence. Women described common expressions of verbal harassment such as: *'bohat patli hai'* (she is too thin), and *'yeh chikni hai'* (she is quite hot). Any reaction or resistance from women practitioners would lead to more humiliating comments such as: *'is liye abhi tak shadi nahi hui'* (this is why she is still a spinster), and *'roz admiyon ke sath kam karke abhi tak akar hai'* (she has chosen to step out of her home and work amongst men in the community, who are not her relatives, and yet she shows attitude).

The language of violence is accompanied with eye contact and restrained gestures such as an attempt to inappropriately touch women practitioners and see how much they can get away with. Pretending to inadvertently touch women and undertake unnecessary examinations were common forms of mild violence. Reporting of verbal harassment is non-existent because the culture has taught women that this is harmless. Also, women are unable to repeat many of the sexual innuendos and shame-inducing language used to demean them at the workplace because it further reduces their status and honour in society. Women are also reluctant to report verbal harassment because they have little faith in the mechanism for deterring perpetrators and also because they fear serious acts of revenge, such as physical abuse or job loss. Clearly, the silent acceptance of verbal violence and the lack of training or inability of women to counter oral aggression contribute to the sustenance of this type of violence. A doctor described the kind of verbal violence faced by women practitioners:

I prefer to drink cold energy drinks rather than tea and coffee.

There is a group of male doctors who are commonly known to snicker and pass comments against women practitioners. Once they very sarcastically called out: 'Is everything OK with you ... why do you need so many energy drinks? How busy were you last night?' Some men don't just use disrespectful innuendos; they are very upfront with their verbal sexual aggression. For example, male colleagues or seniors will approach you with comments like 'Your hair look different today.' If by mistake you answer or smile, it is considered an acceptance of flirtation. Young and inexperienced girls are easily trapped in this way and thereafter will continue to hear more of the same. You have to shut men up very early on by either ignoring them or by not responding to their comments but you have to be very respectful because making enemies of the men is not the solution either. You never know when they will blame you for something.

Another doctor described how it was impossible to report verbal violence, as it meant repeating odious words which only caused a greater loss of honour to women victims:

Verbal violence can never be reported. I'll tell you why ... once I and a female class fellow were sitting in the library when a senior medical officer said some offensive things to us and also revealed his private parts. We were very disturbed and upset and thought of reporting this incident to the principal [of the medical college] or the head of our department but later we dropped the idea. How would we repeat such words and describe what he had done? What if they didn't believe us? What if the medical officer [the perpetrator] lied about us? For example, he could claim that one of us was his girlfriend or ex-girlfriend and we were trying to malign him. Things like this have happened in the past.

## Powerful male networks

Strong male networks in the health sector oblige women victims to accept violence. Male networks make it difficult for women practitioners to survive in the same city or province after reporting violence, as shaming, revenge, and a further infliction of violence follows them from one ward to another or one hospital to another. In many cases women have no choice but to abandon the profession. Most medical specializations in Pakistan are dominated, controlled, and administrated by men.[8] Nurse participants confirmed that they faced more violence in male-dominated wards. It is the dominant representation of men across wards which keep women in subordinate positions with a lower status in the eyes of co-workers and patients. Therefore, in the event of patients and family attendants hearing of a faulty diagnosis or sudden mortality, it is the inferior women practitioners who suffer the impact of violence. A doctor from the surgical ward described the injustices perpetrated by a culture that is inimical to women both in the society and the workplace:

We live in a *sifarish*[9] culture, with mostly men benefiting from the system. Only men benefit from *sifarish* in Pakistan. When we face violence from male perpetrators, we are told to report it to male-dominated administrations or male department heads. How can such a system work? The men always band together and they are able to turn the tables on women victims by squarely placing the blame on them somehow or the other.

A nurse described how women practitioners had to be careful to remain within feminized specialties and departments to avoid violence:

Women practitioners who are trying to compete with their male counterparts in male territories face more of all types of violence in comparison to women within the home. We [women practitioners] are constantly and systematically abused through neglect, discrimination, and humiliation. Women doctors who want to specialize in general surgery are ridiculed and dissuaded. I was told by my professor: 'Isn't it enough to have become a doctor; now you want to become a surgeon too? You should leave that to the men. My daughter specialized in pathology.[10] Choose a specialization more suitable for girls.'

## Licentious male professors

I made a concerted effort to obtain confirmation from women practitioners that they faced violence from male perpetrators, and to ascertain the socio-cultural reasons for men being dominant perpetrators of violence and to understand the reasons for women's acceptance and ownership of male offenders within the community. Individual interview transcripts clearly and uniformly showed that women working in male dominated work organizations suffer from regressive socio-cultural norms putting them at extreme and consistent risk of violence. Of relevance is the fact that women felt angry and disgusted towards certain depraved and licentious senior male healthcare practitioners and administrators who become influential role models for other men in the health sector. Not only do they support the violence perpetrated by their male

team members and subordinates, but some are also known to
have more than one wife, to have affairs, and/or be involved
in aggressive accosting of women colleagues, students, and
patients. There is no social stigma attached to or professional
accountability for licentious senior professors, with the health
community turning a blind eye and indirectly permitting
the continuation of such behaviour. A doctor shared her
experience of facing threats and sexual harassment at the
hands of her senior:

> I was posted to a district headquarter as a medical officer
> during the early years of my career. The district medical
> officer (DMO) there was a vile old man. It was well known
> that a nurse used to supply him with a girl every night at
> his residence. His wife and children lived in another city. I
> used to feel his eyes on me during meetings and I was most
> uncomfortable in his presence. When I discovered that the
> medical staff, with the tacit approval of the DMO, was selling
> the free government-supplied medicines for poor patients in
> the open market, I wrote a complaint to the centre. When the
> DMO learnt about this, he wrote a false report against me
> to the centre telling them that I was habitually late for work
> and did not do my job satisfactorily. Then the threats began
> to come from a junior medical officer (MO). I was warned
> that the local feudal lord was a close friend of the DMO
> and that they would pick me up one day and cause me to
> disappear. It was scary and particularly strange because before
> this occurred, the MO had been very kind and supportive.
> This is just an example of how one corrupt senior officer can
> completely alter the behaviour of the subordinate males in
> his team.

A nurse described the debauched characters of some senior doctors who could not be trusted to afford respect or safety to women practitioners:

> Some of our professors are such bad role models. They have several wives and then also have affairs in the hospitals. We are regularly warned by senior female colleagues not to be too friendly with senior male professors who have bad reputations, as our politeness can be misconstrued. We have heard that once a very corrupt head of department was removed from his post but after the elections, he was reinstated. He then proceeded to take revenge against the women doctors and nurses who had leaked stories about his sexual misdemeanours.

## Security and monitoring

Though it is true that resource and staffing deficiencies in Pakistan's health sector precipitate violence, it cannot be ignored that minimal security and monitoring of violence also plays a significant role in sustaining violence. Aggressive and violent reactions on the part of family members of a patient on hearing the news of his/her demise or terminal illness are an accepted norm in Pakistan, with women practitioners being the easiest targets. In large public sector hospitals with an average daily turnover of 2,000 outpatients and 1,250 inpatients, there are a maximum of only 15–20 guards. Moreover, the few security guards that exist are deployed at the hospital gates to help cars to park, to monitor emergency arrivals, and be visible for VIPs and the media. Women participants suggested that if a larger number of security guards were deployed for their protection, especially in high risk departments such as in the emergency, general medicine, and surgical wards, it would act as a deterrent for perpetrators of violence. A doctor described the deplorable legal and monitoring conditions which encouraged violence:

> All men in our society are violent. Facing violence is a daily routine of our [women healthcare practitioners'] lives. You know why men behave like this? They are not answerable to anyone. There are no laws or accountability. If there was heightened security and easily accessible reporting bodies for women which assured accountability and punishment of perpetrators, things might gradually improve in the hospitals.

An LHW described an incident of being warned, by bullets, to stop participating in the polio immunization drive:

> There is regular street violence against us. We all have schools in our area to cover. My partner LHW and I reached a school one morning to administer anti-polio drops to the students. Thank God the students had already entered the school gates and classes when suddenly we heard motorbikes revving behind us and then the sound of firing. My colleague and I were not fired at directly but they were trying to warn us. Six or seven bullets were fired into the boundary wall of the school. We suspect that community men hire or tip off Pathan (Afghan) men to do such things. They are aggressive and vicious. They would be willing to kill us without a second thought.

## Laws and accountability

The women healthcare practitioners strongly believed that the state and legal system were primarily responsible for the sustenance of violence against women in Pakistan, both at homes and at the workplace. Though harassment laws are being passed, women practitioners complained of the lack of implementation given the complex social norms and beliefs. A web of socio-professional barriers prevents laws from being implemented and women from disclosing violence. These include fears of further damaging the professional status of women workers, being ostracized or fired from male-dominated organizational teams, or being forced by family members to leave the job or even the profession altogether. It was suggested that the only way women would begin to report violence and thereby deter perpetrators was through strong structural support for accountability. Though bodies like the Pakistan Medical and Dental Council and the Health Ministry exist, they have been monopolized for the betterment of the careers of male healthcare practitioners. A staff nurse and a medical officer, who are both actively involved with the local nursing union and the Young Doctors Association, summarized their views:

> Violence by male co-workers, patients, and family attendants is a frequent phenomenon. Recently we [women nurses and doctors in Punjab] went on strike after a staff nurse was beaten up by a senior doctor. However, we had to go back to work in a day or two because otherwise our wages would have been cut. The only way legal or structural policy can be reformed to protect nurses at the workplace is if male public health administration and state officials sincerely believe in the cause.

A nurse-superintendent concluded, in relation to the inefficacy of the existing laws and the social barriers for women in reporting victimization:

A new harassment law has been passed which enables us to report violence to an elected officer and the perpetrator will be punished. But tell me, until society and the mindset changes, how will such laws get implemented? How many women do you think will report harassment? Only a certain type of women dares to report harassment and seek justice: the type who has no fear of retribution and job loss and no family to suffer shame and dishonour! Only laws that suit men and élite families get implemented. Our principal problem is the lack of security and accountability. Everyone in the community knows that they can get away with abusing and threatening us.

## Media projections

The convoluted role of the social media in condoning and creating opportunities for violence were discussed. The women participants revealed that workplace violence directed against them is a culturally accepted phenomenon projected by Pakistan's social media. Daily soaps on local television channels and cinema both depicted everyday violence against women as being justified on the ground of female betrayal of family honour. These female 'misdemeanours' were described by women practitioners as: (1) attempting to gain an education, (2) marrying a man of their own choice, and (3) attempting to pursue an independent career and earn an independent income. Most media storylines imply that the men concerned had no choice other than to inflict violence on the errant women in order to retain their family honour and societal traditions.

Overall, the media has portrayed perpetrators of violence in a heroic light and women victims as deserving of violence which has had a very invidious impact on community attitudes. In addition, the media has always been accustomed to portraying women healthcare practitioners in a bold, audacious, and sexual manner. The sexual objectification of women practitioners (especially nurses and community healthcare providers), through media images, television shows, and literary content has been a contributory factor in encouraging a climate of disrespect for and assignment of an inferior identity to women practitioners. Finally, many women practitioners have become victims of social media-related crimes, such as having their accounts hacked, receiving morphed pictures of themselves on Facebook, getting accosted on WhatsApp, and getting trolled on Twitter or Instagram. Women who covered their hair and faces at the workplace were not victimized as much in this way, and many participants believed that their liberal attire was an encouragement to cyber predators. Participants described how they not only felt unsafe posting pictures to friends but that they were also scared of emailing personal details and documents relating to important matters. Many felt that joining the workforce had left them with little privacy and anonymity in the community. A staff nurse highlighted stereotypes created by local media through the representation of women practitioners as either victims or seductive sirens:

> The most familiar themes of popular local dramas revolve around violence against women. In the dramas women who get abused most frequently are those who are independent and work outside the home. Besides, women practitioners have been depicted by the media as beautiful and tempting seductresses who save the lives of men and then promptly fall in love with them. That is why patients say the most inappropriate

things, like: 'I have become ill in order to be saved by you' and 'It was my fantasy to be taken care of by you.'

A doctor described the negative consequences at the workplace caused by sexual objectification of women practitioners:

As you know, nurses and women doctors have always been projected as sexual objects through media and literature. This harms us in our work life. I will give you one example of this. There was a Facebook group created by our male colleagues where they used to post pictures of female colleagues taken from different angles. They morphed our pictures and pasted our faces on pornographic body images with disgusting captions. These pictures were purposely leaked to cause embarrassment and humiliation amongst the women. Perhaps they were sending a message to the women who were not covering their heads that this is what could be done to them. I was very scared that my picture would be used for such a purpose. I had no way of finding out. I have since deleted my old Facebook account and created a new one, with only members of my immediate family and some women friends added as 'Friends'. I do not post my pictures anymore and regularly change my passwords.

## Religious misinterpretation

Most of the women healthcare practitioners discussed that religious authorities and local Imams[11] exercised great power over public opinion, and more particularly over the male population of the region. Practitioners described how religion is misrepresented by being taken out of context and propagated to gullible and illiterate masses. Women suffer sustained violence due to misinterpretation by religious authorities who provide men in the community with the sanction to perpetrate violence against women. It was revealed how religious leaders within the community were generally violent against LHWs and their own female family members. Once violence is perpetrated by religious leaders, such behaviour becomes the approved norm for other men in the community. Unfortunately, there is no central religious authority in Pakistan to register such problems. Too many religious sects and theological bodies would need to be approached in order to help to holistically alter cultural attitudes and religious misinterpretations. A doctor elaborated on how perpetrators of workplace violence did not consider their actions to be wrong but rather believed that they were helping to keep women in their 'proper position':

It was a busy day in the ICU and no doctors were available. I and two staff nurses were attempting to handle the patients. One of the family attendants hit the back of my head and manhandled me into checking a relative of his. I asked him to stop and enquired: 'Don't you have a mother or a sister at home?' To this he responded, 'Of course I do, and that is why I know how to make you do your duty. Islam has commanded us to guide our women.'

An LHW described her experience with the local religious leader in the community she served:

It is not in the power of women to change the culture and beliefs of the community. It is the elders and the maulanas[12] who control all this. There is a local maulana who consistently prevents us from administering polio drops to his six children. He claims, 'There are no children in this house.' Once I got really frustrated by his tone and vulgar leer and responded, 'May Allah punish the liars as befits Him.' The furious maulana brought some of his students from the masjid, tall and aggressive ones, to our BHU centre and threatened that if any 'immoral' and 'shameless' LHWs were sent to his house in the future, he would not be responsible for what happened to them. It was a direct physical threat against us. We knew how these men beat their wives and were aware that they would not think twice about treating us in the same way. Imams and maulanas of the community expect us to passively accept violence, and God forbid if we ever stand up for ourselves, they turn into even greater monsters. That is because they think they have God on their side.

## Conclusion

In the light of the wide range and diverse causes of workplace violence directed against women healthcare practitioners, it becomes evident that women in Pakistan are struggling against major cultural and structural forces that sustain and encourage violence. The struggle for increased safety and protection for women practitioners attempts to challenge age-old traditions of patriarchy, culture, history, and superstition. The social construction of gender roles and community interests bolster low professional status and negative identity for women practitioners. Professional bullying and verbal harassment are commonly employed to humiliate and defame women. Men have proven themselves to be powerful perpetrators who have reduced laws and accountability systems to ineffective levels across organizations and communities where care provision exists. The VIP culture, media representation, and class stratification in Pakistan further contributes to the physical and sexual victimization of women. Sadly, a large section of the public considers women practitioners to be immoral and/or unreligious and this contributes to the transgressions. Unless the momentous socio-religious barriers preventing the reporting of violence are eliminated, perpetrators will have free reign to continue with their violent and nefarious acts.

## NOTES

1. The booking of interview times was scheduled either with an early breakfast or a lunch. Although this placed a strain on the personal funds I had allocated to my research project, it helped to secure a sense of easy camaraderie with the women healthcare practitioners and provided the latter with an additional incentive to provide some free time for the interviews in the midst of a hectic and challenging schedule both at work and at home.
2. Ethnic harassment includes discrimination based on race, creed, religious belief, and both provincial and regional belonging.
3. Nihari is a South Asian meat curry consisting of beef or lamb along with bone marrow. It is considered a prestigious national dish and is commonly available from local food vendors as a takeaway meal to be eaten with local bread or naan.
4. Street violence and frequent crossfire is not uncommon in the region.
5. Haram translates into earning of money from an illegitimate or illegal source.
6. A *dupatta* is an additional free-flowing piece of material worn by women in the country, approximately three metres long, which is wrapped loosely across the shoulders and the chest. The top usually starts from the neck and ends near the knees and thighs. It can be easily stripped off a woman, unlike a pinned head scarf or a burqa gown that covers the full body and has sleeves.

7. *Saab* translates as 'Sir' in English. It is an honorific used to address senior males at the workplace and in educational institutes.

8. The male-dominated medical professions include, amongst others, the departments of accident and emergency, cardiology, general medicine and surgery, orthopaedics, nephrology, oncology, gastroenterology, ophthalmology, dermatology, and neurosurgery.

9. *Sifarish* is an urdu word which describes the accepted culture of achieving aims and avoiding formal procedures by pulling off strings, using influential contacts to get a job done via bribery or nepotism.

10. Pathology is a specialty that deals with lab work. It is considered suitable for Pakistani women given the conservative belief that it will restrict women to the lab and thereby limit interaction with men in the clinical areas.

11. Imams are considered religious authorities who not only lead the compulsory congregational prayers five times a day in the local mosque but also deliver Friday sermons and have considerable influence over the beliefs and actions of the community, especially over men.

12. Maulanas are local religious instructors, under whom students are taught to read and memorize the Quran. Local maulanas are usually able to read Arabic or have memorized the Quran by heart. The majority are however untrained and unversed in the actual meaning of the Quran given an inability to understand the Arabic language, or to distinguish between the literal and the metaphorical.

# 5

# Women Practitioners
# in Support of Cyclical Violence

Although women in Pakistan are taught from birth not to discuss issues relating to abuse, I was extremely satisfied with the grounded, qualitative accounts that emerged from the interviews. Perhaps the women practitioners felt a need to share their experiences with a non-judgemental and sympathetic female confidante. This chapter discusses the wider social constructs of socio-economic liabilities which submerge women practitioners in a cycle of victimization and their own roles in their sustained oppression. Measures for women's emancipation are usually linked to work participation and an ability to earn an independent income. However, in Pakistan, women's education and economic involvement is more dependent on male authority and decision-making. Men control which professions women join and their treatment at the workplace. Women remain silent spectators unable and unwilling to communicate to the world and each other about their workplace conditions and challenges. Educated and working women, more than the uneducated and unemployed, are to blame for accepting victimization so passively. Although the women practitioners shared clandestine accounts about adopting secrecy patterns and owning that they had been victims of perpetrators, the majority were unwilling to admit that they too were responsible for the sustained workplace violence against their own gender. The blame was shifted to cultural conditioning, upbringing, and rigid social expectations. Some of the senior women doctors who read my findings agreed that this area needed to be placed in the forefront of my research to drive home to women practitioners that much of their oppression stems from their own failures and inaction.

## Forced Professions and Conflict amongst Women Practitioners

In poor and conservative countries like Pakistan, many women are reluctantly permitted to engage in out-of-home work participation through financial necessity. Women practitioners, including nurses, LHWs, and doctors from the lower socio-economic strata are under great pressure to remain in the profession notwithstanding unfavourable work organizations and a lack of safety. The social respect attributed to lower-class women practitioners working to supplement household income is lesser than the respect afforded to upper-class women doctors who work by choice. Lower-class practitioners face greater violence because the perpetrators believe such women, under compulsion to retain their jobs, will not resist or report violence. Women suffer from contradictory family forces which explicitly ban them from working outside the home and yet covertly grant them permission to do so (due to financial necessity). As overt social approval is not common, it leaves women practitioners exposed to sustained shaming and disparagement by extended family members and the community. A married LHS described the slander she faced from the community and the consequent anxiety she felt for the reputation of her parents and children:

> My family was against me joining the profession but there was a vacancy and I applied. Everyone was happy when my first pay cheque came. It was necessary to contribute to the family income. When I got married, my in-laws refused to let me work. My mother in law was accusatory: 'Your mother worked a spell of black magic on me and got me to choose an immoral LHW like you who assists women to have abortions!' My husband's job and income was irregular and he eventually allowed me to resume my job. It is for the sake of money that I have to hear abuse, not just against myself, but against my parents too and this I can barely stand. If it was not for the money I would leave the profession again, as I know that the slander of the community and my in-laws hurts my children.

A staff nurse shared the burden of having to work due to financial necessity:

> It has become necessary for women to leave the house to earn money. Our men [father, brother, husband] pretend not to like it in the presence of the larger family and elders but in private they encourage us. The perpetrators of violence are aware that because of their financial needs, women cannot leave their jobs and that is why they continue with their abusive ways. Rich women doctors are respected by society because they are viewed to be working due to their skills and not for money.

Respect and honour for Pakistani families is tied to receiving timely and respectable proposals for their daughters.

The acceptable order for arranged marriages is that proposals are received from the groom's family. A woman who does not receive an arranged marriage proposal from a suitable family and instead enters into a love marriage through personal choice is shamed in society for being 'immoral' and 'degenerate'. Even when a man initiates the proposal to a woman of his choice, after studying or working with her, the community norm is to blame the woman for having 'trapped' or 'seduced' the man. Due to this social understanding, participant mothers with daughters described how they felt the pressure of maintaining their social standing in the community to enable their daughters to receive good marriage proposals.

One way of securing a good marriage proposal for daughters is by forcing them to study medicine which is a high status degree for women in Pakistan, and much sought after in the marriage market. As greater shaming and harassment is reserved for single women, society rigidly conforms to the social requirements of the marriage market. Many mothers confessed that they did not want to leave their daughters unmarried in a society such as that in Pakistan which victimizes single women. The problems that arise in treating medical degrees for women as marriage tickets are substantial. Equating these as such and then immediately going on to marry and bear children devalues the academic resources and socio-economic impact of female work participation. It is also true that many women are being socially compelled to enter a profession that may not have been their primary choice, and then prohibited from practising it in order to assume socially sanctioned domestic roles.

Not only are women being victimized by getting robbed off of the right to make their own life choices but in the event that women doctors choose to practise medicine, they become more vulnerable to bullying and abuse from the family, in-laws, and the community at large. This is because woman doctors begin to rapidly lose their social status when engaging in out-of-home clinical work. Male doctors who shoulder a greater responsibility in recognizing the value of their women colleagues are also reluctant to marry women practitioners. There is the fear that by assuming responsibility and control in a hectic vocation like medicine, women will not be able to perform their primary responsibilities of marriage, home management, and reproduction. Families and in-laws are especially reluctant to let women practise in the health sector because it entails care provision, leaving less energy and emotional care for the home. A doctor described how she was coerced into the medical profession by her family:

I remember my mother lecturing me after my Matric exam (I was then only 15 years old) that medicine was the only noble and socially acceptable profession for girls. My parents wanted me to get enrolled for the FSc pre-medical and they hoped that before I completed my final year medical exams, I would be engaged. Good proposals are easier to come by for girls who are medical students. I was too young to refuse and too scared at the thought of not receiving a timely wedding proposal. In our country most women medical students have been forced, overtly or covertly, to become doctors. I now understand that as a medical student, I and others like me were frustrated and stressed at having been coerced into this profession. We did not look forward to the long years of study and difficult exams. Our mental stress was compounded by having to suffer through the nasty ways and bullying of male colleagues and seniors.

Another doctor shared her anguish at the treatment of single working women practitioners in the community and at the workplace:

I am 29 years old and have been working in the hospital for many years now. I am still single and perhaps past the age of receiving proposals. As you know, in Pakistan, girls above the age of 25 do not receive arranged marriage proposals. A match-making aunty comes regularly to our house. She takes a monthly stipend for her efforts but brings very bad proposals. I heard her tell my mother, 'Why did you let your daughter work at the hospital? Families prefer girls who have studied medicine but are not practising it.' Because I am not married, I regularly encounter sneers, jibes, name-calling, and sexual taunts at the hospital. Life for single women is very tough in our society, and that is why Pakistani parents want to get their daughters married on time.

A nurse described how practising in the medical and nursing profession lowered the prospects of many women practitioners to receive an attractive proposal:

The male house officers and medical officers will do their utmost to inveigle us into a relationship, use us, perhaps even sleep with us, and then discard us. A majority of them will never consider marrying us. They will consider marriage with younger girls who have studied at women's colleges and graduated in subjects such as home economics or literature. Such girls come from traditional backgrounds, are less exposed, and more sheltered which makes them appear more attractive. They might also consider marriage with women medical students but rarely with women nurses and doctors who have begun practising in the clinic.

Women healthcare practitioners share very little solidarity and unity in comparison to their male counterparts in the country with a weak and fragmented union movement. Notwithstanding regular strikes and demonstrations, the efforts of the nursing and young doctors' associations across Punjab and Sindh have been unable to achieve anything in terms of structured improvement on women's safety issues. Indeed, most of the protests organized by the nursing and doctor unions have been directed towards adequate compensation and service structure rather than issues of harassment and violence. The principal reasons for this inability to formally and strategically coordinate efforts on issues of violence and safety are: (1) the heavy workload at home and at work, and a consequent lack of time, and (2) the absence of women leaders in the health sector. However, another fundamental factor contributes to undermining women practitioner unity and mutual respect. A majority of LHWs believe that many women nurses who do not work in their own domicile and live in hospital accommodation take advantage of being away from their families and engage in affairs with male doctors. Most of the doctor participants corroborated the LHW claims about nurses and also added that the latter had fewer opportunities for developing illegitimate relationships or dalliances because they worked in the neighbourhood in which they lived.

Regrettably it is not just the male members of society who are guilty of victim-blaming. A deeply regressive conflict exists in terms of women doctors and LHWs viewing female nurses as being immoral and licentious. It was suggested by LHWs and women doctors that society tends to generalize the negative labels of nurses on other women practitioners, contributing to the sustenance of violence. Many women doctors and LHWs believe themselves to be victims because of the behaviour of their 'sinful' nurse counterparts. Women nurses, in turn, believe that women doctors have greater influence and status, but find it demeaning to join hands with nurses, and therefore the cause of gender equality and safety for women practitioners in the health sector suffers overall. The blame game between women practitioners in relation to their inferior status prevents them from becoming a team which could effectively mobilize for workplace safety. A woman doctor explained why it was important for the reputation of women doctors to keep a distance from women nurses:

It is a certain breed of women nurses that mixes loosely with male doctors and have affairs with them. We have seen nurses in rooms doing all sorts of things with doctors. They [nurses] are more prone to acting in this way. One of the reasons for their [nurses] embroilment in licentious affairs is because they join after Matric [are are only 16 to 18 years of age] and thus are more vulnerable to sweet talk and false promises. It is the nurses overall who have managed to ruin the reputation of all other women practitioners and have made working life very difficult for us. Nurses never waste any opportunity to undermine and make trouble for us (women doctors) in the hospital. We try to stay away from them and our social circles at the workplace are not the same.

Another doctor described a specific incident relating to the known transgressions of women nurses:

We suffer sexual harassment regularly. This is because of

the bad reputations and misdeeds of a few nurses. I have come across nurses who are having affairs with doctors. My nephew once had to be taken to the hospital due to severe dehydration. I went to look for the nurse on night duty to ask her to administer the drip. As she was not at the nursing desk I looked inside some of the office rooms and finally found her. She was with a male doctor in a very compromising position. I was shocked and upset. She saw me and followed me down. She gave my nephew a drip and then gestured to me. She wanted to talk to me privately, probably to ask me not to tell anyone, but I did not respond as I wanted nothing to do with her.

An LHW explained one of the reasons for the 'lack of morals' among women nurses:

Nurses move from district to district without roots and have affairs with any doctors and influential men they can get their hands on. We LHWs belong to the community and we have roots here. We do not deserve the bad reputation with which all women practitioners are labelled because of nurses. We are not like them.

## Accepting Violence and Owning Perpetrators

Women healthcare practitioners, especially nurses and LHWs, are front line practitioners in the hospital setting and at the doorsteps of the community. This makes them easy targets for assault and more vulnerable victims of violence in stressful and precarious settings. Both public sector organizations and slum areas where women healthcare practitioners are working have frustrated and agitated men who are known to take out their aggressions on women. Similarly, women physiotherapists are undermined and humiliated by the community by being labelled 'masseurs'. This is a dehumanizing experience for women providers who have to remain geographically mobile in the community and are dependent on the public extending to them honour and respect for the responsibilities they undertake. The absence of manifest protection by the state to community workers and the knowledge of regular but unsuccessful strikes for increased security by LHWs is a further invitation to perpetrators to continue their violence without fear of accountability. A nurse described the vulnerable position of front line practitioners:

> Doctors do their rounds and go away. We nurses are front line practitioners who spend more time at the hospital and have greater interaction with patients. We are easy targets for abuse. As doctors become senior they devote most of their time to their private practices. There are some senior professors and department heads who visit the hospital only once a week, and others who visit even less frequently than that. Their team of doctors and assistant professors, and even the principal, cover for them. That is how government money is wasted and patients are neglected. The absence of even a single doctor or surgeon results in major delays in the care delivery to patients, causing them to justifiably become violent. This violence can only be taken out on women staff and nurses, as we are the most visible and also the people who cannot retaliate.

A woman physiotherapist, who visits clients at their homes in the evening after hospital shifts, shared her experience:

When we visit homes, we regularly hear family members or servants call out, 'Oh the massage lady has come'. We are used to this now, but on one occasion a very upsetting incident took place. I charge PKR 800[1] for a single therapy session for patients who cannot come to the hospital. Each session lasts about 45–60 minutes. On a regular visit to a woman client, the husband opened the gate and invited me in, saying, 'Come in, my wife is inside'. He slid open the bolt of the gate and went inside the house, only to return a few seconds later. He confirmed what I had suspected, 'My wife is not home but I wanted to ask you something important. I heard how much you earn in a day and I felt really bad for you and your colleagues. I wanted to share a job with you that could help you to earn much more money.' Very reluctantly, I asked, 'What kind of job, Brother?' He said, 'I work in the film industry. You and your colleagues can come there and give the men massages. Other women perform these services too but they are not trained like you.' I backed away and quickly fled the house, exclaiming, 'Brother, thank you, but I have to go home now!' I never related this incident to anyone, especially to family members. I accepted the incident to be my fault and now I ensure to call and re-check if the client is home for the appointment just before I set off to see them.

It is perhaps the son-worshipping culture which places men on pedestals and sanctifies their actions, forcing women victims to accept blame for assaults against them. Deviant behaviour of men is sanctified not just by social laws and religious misinterpretation but also by organizational structures. Cultural laws of the organization, the hidden curriculum in the health sector, and a male administration combine to exert immense pressure on women practitioners never to defame male perpetrators by reporting violence. Women healthcare practitioners, and especially nurses and LHWs, have such a low status in Pakistani society that they accept the superior status of the perpetrators and justify their actions because they fear that by reacting adversely they will create more professional and personal trouble for themselves in the process of seeking retribution. A nurse described the process of owning perpetrators and forgiving them rather than deterring them through punishment:

Recently there was a doctor who was sexually harassing a number of women staff members. The nurses went on strike and because the newspapers picked up the story, the health minister got involved. Top officials and our health administration coerced us to forgive the perpetrator and that was the end of the story. We were repeatedly told this was the only way for us to retain our self-respect. There is no penalization for male perpetrators, only forgiveness and acceptance.

An LHW described how women practitioners focused on avoiding violence rather than putting a stop to it:

We have to create a family register of the territory to which we are assigned, which is around 200–250 families. This is difficult for us because many families reject us and label us as outsiders. We are considered enemies of the community who are attempting to destroy the traditions of society through our services and this is why we face so much violence. I cannot tell you about the *rangbarang-thashadud*[2] we face but we accept all of this. After all, members of our own extended family do not accept us. We liken the community to our extended family.

If we accept the abuse and disrespect of our relatives, why shouldn't we accept the behaviour of the rest of the community too? There is no alternative to acceptance.

Another LHW described how women practitioners felt obliged to accept perpetrators from their community:

My sister-in-law and I became LHWs together. At the time we were unaware that the profession was likened to prostitution. When we pass through the neighbourhood, men on the streets such as roadside cobblers or food vendors, who are aware of our profession, call out to us offensively for sexual favours. We do not feel safe walking along these streets alone, and especially at night. We don't resist or raise our voices and just accept it. This is because we are part of the community and have to tolerate such behaviour. These are our men after all.

## The Hidden Pact

Women participants revealed another grave problem in Pakistan's public hospitals relating to violence against women patients. It is not just women practitioners who suffer from the lack of security, monitoring, and violence but also women patients from poor and illiterate backgrounds. The participants explained that women patients are at a higher risk of unnecessary examination and assault, especially in isolated operation theatres and in private rooms. Alarmingly, not just male co-workers but men from their community were also cited as common perpetrators of violence against women patients. Family members and acquaintances who were aware that women were alone and isolated in the hospital were able to perpetrate all types of violence such as visiting them without their consent, verbally and psychologically harassing them, or even raping patients confined to bed.

The interviews revealed that women practitioners who had to silently witness violence against women patients and also assist women victims at the workplace, suffered immense psychological strain and anxiety. Working with abusive male practitioner perpetrators who are not being held accountable for their actions is a constant source of apprehension and stress for women practitioners even when they are not direct victims themselves. Women described how they were required, as part of their job, to remain emotionally unattached but that they were unable to do so due to continuing fears of either having to witness violence or having to face it themselves. A doctor described how male practitioners often took advantage of the proximity and position of women patients to sexually exploit them in the hospital:

Frustrated male doctors and staff will not waste an opportunity to sensually touch the bodies of women patients. Unnecessary and repeated examinations of the chest area for thyroid and breast surgery patients are common. During surgery, women patients are completely vulnerable. The male doctors have access to every part of the body. They are known to explore the female genitalia, the legs, and the rest. We know about this but cannot do anything. Many senior doctors unnecessarily compel young women doctors to undertake genital examinations of male patients and then talk indecently to them during or after examination. It is not that other doctors may not be doing this abroad but like my cousin who works in Houston tells me, there are anonymous and transparent reporting bodies within the hospital to deal with such issues and punish repeat offenders. We have no such reprieve. Because of incidents like this and the failure to be able to protect ourselves and women patients, we are under a lot of stress and guilt.

A nurse shared the extreme mistrust and disdain women practitioners felt for depraved male doctors:

We do not respect or trust the doctors in our community. You cannot imagine the things we know about them. Once a poor woman was taken for an emergency C-section and the male surgeon misbehaved with the poor woman. She was unconscious and was made to remain unconscious for longer than necessary. When she came out from the operation theatre, her mother asked, 'What are these bite marks on her face and neck; what has happened to our daughter?' Such a shameful society we live in, where we cannot even trust male doctors. The public considers male doctors to be like gods.

Another woman doctor described the lack of security and protection for female patients in public hospitals:

Recently there was a girl patient [studying in the tenth grade] admitted to the hospital. A boy from her class sneaked into the hospital and raped her. How do things like this happen? People can just sneak into our hospital and do all kinds of things which is a great failure of our public hospitals. We have heard of other cases where family members or community members rape and abuse women patients in the vicinity of the hospital but we have to remain silent because the women and their families do not want to report such incidents.

Pakistan still comprises a large majority of silent housewives, who are victims of domestic violence. Family members and in-laws are known to perpetrate collective violence against women within the homes to control their life decisions relating to education, social mobility, marriage, family size, child immunization, and work participation. Most women healthcare practitioners confirmed that they came across, both in the hospital and in the field, a considerable number of women patients who had suffered from domestic violence. Women patients almost always lied to the practitioners about the reasons for their injuries for fear of dishonour, social ostracization, and retribution. Although women practitioners are able to recognize cases of domestic abuse which are not reported, they support women of the community to 'suffer silently' and keep incidents of violence they encounter a secret. It is an accepted cultural norm, for both women healthcare practitioners facing workplace violence and female patients visiting the hospital due to injuries from domestic violence, to 'never' report violence.

The role of women practitioners as female conspirators in keeping domestic violence a secret was justified by arguing that disclosure for Pakistani women, especially those from disadvantaged backgrounds, only led to greater suffering through revenge on the part of the husband and in-laws, retribution on the children, and the possibility of divorce. For women from underprivileged and conservative families it is always better to embrace violence silently, as families are reluctant to support daughters when they return home after separation given the financial cost and social disgrace this entails.

Grass roots experiences were used by LHWs to describe the great neglect of women in Pakistani society. Women are scared of declaring their illnesses or health needs as traditional norms and society have socialized them to believe that only sinful and irreverent women suffer from health adversities and infertility. Strong women of the past who never visited hospitals or sought help from medical practitioners are commonly cited as role models to young women and girls in the community. Therefore, women are ashamed to inquire about health-related issues such as gynaecological abnormalities, pregnancy ailments, and other health problems from trained practitioners. That is why most women in the Pakistan clandestinely seek the services of unskilled traditional healers who are discreetly available within the community. Women found to have taken assistance from LHWs face verbal threats and physical abuse. A staff nurse shared the justifications for women remaining silent after facing domestic violence:

> If a woman patient does not want to acknowledge that her injuries are due to domestic violence, there are usually sound reasons for her silence. Reporting the abuse will in most cases lead to serious retribution. She will most probably end up facing greater violence; her husband could divorce her and take the children away. The legal system and wider society, including her blood relatives, will not support a woman in such situations either. So we [women healthcare practitioners] usually remain silent when we suspect cases of domestic violence where women patients are not willing to tell us what really happened. The best way of supporting them [women patients] is by respecting their privacy and ensuring that they have a home to return to.

An LHW shared the difficulty in providing services to women in the community due to threats and pressure from their husbands and in-laws:

Most of the men from the neighbourhoods we visit use domestic abuse to control their women and vent their frustrations. The women [from the community] do not want us to know about the domestic abuse that they face, and this is also why they avoid us. They [women of the community] are afraid that using our [LHW] services will rob them off of whatever status they have left [in the family and community] and also expose them to greater violence. Once I was begging a husband to take his wife to the hospital for her delivery as there were obvious complications and risks to delivering the child at home with a TBA [traditional birth attendant]. The husband became verbally abusive with me and slapped his heavily pregnant wife to stop her from pleading with him to take my advice. I apologized to him and tried to calm him down for the sake of his wife. We ultimately have to leave such women in the hands of God. If we make a big deal of such incidents we will be permanently banned from the community.

As very few women want to admit to experiencing violence, it means that the actual prevalence of violence is difficult to measure in a country like Pakistan. Women participants confirmed that there is a hidden and unspoken pact amongst women co-workers and patients in the health sector to avoid reporting both workplace and domestic violence. Interviews revealed that as daughters, sisters, and mothers, women were most afraid of jeopardizing their family honour and respect in the community. The families of victims have to suffer the shame of hearing that their women have become 'impure' or worst of all that their debauchery had invited victimization. The gravest risk for women of reporting violence was that society almost invariably categorized daughters in the same way as their mothers and participants insisted that many women would not report abuse in order to protect the reputation of their daughters. A doctor described the dilemma of disclosure:

> Remaining silent is in our favour because reporting violence only ruins our reputation and the team dynamics in the hospital. The victims are labelled troublemakers and no one wants to work with them. Senior male professors have been known to get victims transferred to other departments or have them altogether blacklisted from the hospital.

A nurse went on to elaborate on the negative impact of reporting violence, especially on the families of women practitioners:

> We [women healthcare practitioners] have a silent pact never to report victimization. We try to push the memories of abuse and beatings, the language, and the behaviour to the back of our minds and not talk about it much. It is not something we can even think of discussing with our families, husband, sons, children, or in-laws. Perhaps they are vaguely aware of it as the media highlights the plight of nurses but we cannot reveal the details. We cannot share our shame with them. They will also be shamed if they are aware of the conditions in which we work. It is very bad, especially for our daughters, if the family and relatives find out the details of our experience with workplace violence.

## Coping Strategies against Violence

The women participants were asked what coping strategies they had adopted, if any, in a work culture which did not provide them structural and cultural protection against violence. The strategies used to cope with aggression and abuse included partial care delivery, desultory work commitment, and engaging in lies and deception. Interestingly, the participants also described the adoption of superficial characteristics of being sullen, aloof, reserved, and harried in order to deter people from engaging in superfluous conversation and permitting minimal interaction. The women admitted that they did feel guilty for delivering partial care or intervention on behalf of the patients but that this was necessary to ensure their protection in the current work environment. This was a disturbing discovery given that retraction of teamwork, care-provision, and error-reporting has profoundly negative influences on recovery and mortality in public health.

The chief underlying learning during clinical practice for women practitioners is that of protecting themselves from doctors, patients, and family attendants, and remaining vigilant at all times. In the process of having to deal with personal safety before patient-safety, women practitioners not only face great mental strain but they bear a heavy invisible work burden for which they are not compensated. To mitigate violence, women also attempt to remain aware of the likely precipitators of workplace violence, such as, a large number of family attendants, busy wards, expected death or unfavourable diagnosis, and male co-workers of ill-repute. It is expected that women practitioners have a deeper understanding of the need of health-seeking behaviours and counselling after experiencing violence. However, women practitioners are not seeking such assistance either. Instead, they are internalizing their experiences of violence for fear of bringing shame upon themselves. An LHW shared how women practitioners learn to secure their own safety by withdrawing services:

> One of my initial experiences of trying to explain to a father about the importance of giving his child polio drops at his doorstep resulted in him pushing me and kicking my medicine box. We [LHWs] learn very quickly to sense danger and we learn to safeguard ourselves by backing away. We are able to tell from their initial tones and expressions that violence is imminent. Now if a man opens the door and shows reluctance to let me administer polio drops, I back away and do not wait to ask why.

A nurse described the difficulty of implementing in practice the theoretical knowledge of dealing with victimization:

> Men are born with an inclination to perpetrate violence against women. We cannot simultaneously provide care services for others and be on the guard to prevent violence against ourselves. We do not even have the time or energy to share our burdens and fears with female co-workers. We realize that as victims we need counselling and medical help but we avoid this too, largely because we have no time, but also because it will only cause us more complications and shame.

Symbolic precipitators of violence were described, which helped women adopt defensive mechanisms of partial delivery at the workplace, including: (1) the politics of name-calling, and (2) the practitioner uniform. Respectful and derogatory name-calling in the hospital setting is a noticeable feature of Pakistani society. Women practitioners are generally referred to by patients, family attendants, and co-workers as 'nurse' or 'lady doctor'. Participants described how when the honorific 'nurse' is used, it is connoted as a derogatory professional status and coupled with tones of aggression and disrespect, or worst, presumptuousness and imperiousness. Alternatively, when patients, family attendants, and co-workers seek to treat the nurse with respect, they refer to her as: 'sister', *bibi* (madam), *memsab* (madam), *behan* (sister), *baji* (sister), 'madam', or 'mother', and this in a respectful tone.

It was discussed that the use of the term 'lady doctor' by the public to refer to women doctors implies the absence of specialized skill and worth of the practitioner concerned. It is used as a generic term for the necessary inclusion of women in the health sector due to the demands of segregation. Derivatively, women doctors or 'lady doctors' are expected to be solely serving women patients in the gynaecology or maternity departments. There is little or no recognition of women doctors in other specialties. Many participants described how it was common for families to reject the services of women doctors in male-dominated fields such as cardiology, oncology, orthopaedics, and surgery in general. A doctor questioned the honorific used for women doctors:

> Have you ever wondered why male doctors are called just doctor or doctor *saab* (sir), whereas we [women doctors] are called lady doctor? This is to make it clear to us that we have been accepted in this profession to care for female patients alone. 'Lady Doctor' implies that we are not recognized as equal to male doctors and are accepted only to practise in the medical fields of gynaecology and maternity.

The superior status of the doctor's coat as opposed to the inferior symbolic status of the nurse uniform was elaborated upon. Whereas the doctor's coat invited greater esteem and respect, the nurse's uniform attracts lower respect and provides an opening for maltreatment. Easily identifiable nurse uniforms attract negative connotations both at the workplace and in public zones, prompting perpetrators to attack their wearers. Public spaces where violence is regularly practised against nurses in uniform were listed as bus stands, buses, rickshaws, retail shops, fruit vendors, and isolated roads. That is why women practitioners, like nurses and LHWs, who use public transport, shroud themselves in burqas[3] and veil their faces before entering communal zones. A nurse ward-head described the difference in social identity between women doctors and women nurses:

> Women doctors are respected in our society but women nurses are not. Our families are ashamed to tell acquaintances that their daughter is just a 'nurse'. At the workplace when we are called 'sister' [by a co-worker, patient, family attendant, medical student, or a service provider such as a pharmacist], it almost always implies that the person interacting with us is going to behave in a professional, polite, and deferential manner. On the other hand, when we are called 'nurse', it almost invariably means we are going to be dealt with in an abusive and condescending manner.

A young staff nurse described how the nurse uniform is shrouded in public spaces in order to deter violence:

> Student nurses who have left for home in a rush in their uniforms and not heeded the advice of experienced nurses have learnt the hard way by being accosted and stalked by men in public areas. Sadly, our uniform is an indicator for men in

public zones, attracting lecherous glances, physical contact, and sexual overtures. That is why we change from our uniforms into everyday clothes before leaving the hospital, and why we wear the burqa [garment enveloping full-body] and hijab [head scarf]. They are worn to provide us with additional protection.

## Conclusion

The debate about means to end workplace violence against women usually centres on creating deterrence for perpetrators and securing the organizational structure. However, because many women practitioners work in public spaces and the causes of violence have their roots in cultural traditions, there needs to be an enhanced effort to understand victim liabilities. Crippling self-imposed factors cause women practitioners to suffer repeated violence and precludes them from being recipients of secondary and tertiary levels of prevention.[4] Women from the upper and middle classes who have the means and educational background are encouraged to enter the higher status levels of the medical profession, whereas women from the lower classes, through financial necessity, become nurses and LHWs, notwithstanding their lower status and negative identity. Inherent conflicts between women practitioners exist, causing them to remain disunited and uncooperative in collectively spearheading a movement for their personal development and safety. As women begin to accept violence from perpetrators, they ironically have formed a strong invisible pact which conceals incidents of violence and remains silent in the face of offence. Although women practitioners are aware of other women in their community suffering from violence, they prefer to support concealment in order to retain a perception of collective honour and position in society. Women victims have not remained without defence mechanisms to deal with the onslaught of violence. They have developed an ability to sense a precipitation of violence and have adopted partial care delivery in face of events such as specific name-calling, discrimination or harassment due to type of practitioner uniform worn, and/ or high risk emergencies. Women practitioners (including Christians and Hindu nurses) have also turned to using the veil as a form of religious protection against violence. Unfortunately, combating violence with coping strategies of partial care has rendered victims at even greater risk of violence due to inefficient services and has also compromised the patient safety standards in Pakistan. It would not be wrong to conclude that victimization of women practitioners has led to immeasurable socio-financial and health costs for the people of Pakistan.

## NOTES

1. According to conversion rates, as at 12 December 2015, PKR 800 was equivalent to USD 7.65.
2. *Rangbarang-thashadud* literally translates as 'various shades of violence'. The participants interviewed are implying that women face sustained violence of a myriad kind. Women in the healthcare sector perforce accept the many types of violence to which they are subjected, including verbal and physical abuse, professional bullying, and sexual harassment as normal, and are somewhat confused as to how to specifically describe them given the absence of open discussion and education about violence within the community.
3. A burqa is a loosely fitted garment used to cover the full female figure from head to toe, and is commonly black to allow no part of the physical form to be revealed.
4. There are three stages involved in the prevention of violence and

facilitation of victims: (1) primary prevention refers to activities that prevent violence from occurring in the first place, (2) secondary prevention refers to the immediate response after violence to assist the victim in dealing with the short-term consequences of violence, and (3) tertiary prevention refers to long-term response after violence to assist the victim in dealing with the lasting consequences of violence.

# 6

# The Perpetrators' Silent Allies

Women practitioner respondents tended to label all men in general as perpetrators because they tended to consider all passive male bystanders to be equally responsible for the prevalence of violence. That is why the attempt to understand the reasons for and sustenance of workplace violence against women practitioners would be incomplete without listening to the voices of male colleagues. Male practitioners are also the most immediate witnesses to workplace violence against women in the health sector. I found that the male administrative heads in the health sector of the country were very reluctant to discuss issues relating to violence faced by women. Expectedly, it was not that easy to obtain consent to interview male practitioners. Men were reluctant to share their perceptions about violence faced by women co-workers, and some even believed that there was no significant issue of violence against women practitioners in Pakistan. It emerged that a tribal brotherhood is operational across health organizations on the basis of which male perpetrators and male bystanders have together joined to perpetrate and ignore ritual violence against women. This male network is also utilized and effectively directed towards maintaining power and operational authority at the workplace.

In all, through snowball and purposeful sampling, an effort

was made to interview 23 male practitioners from different designations across public sector hospitals of Punjab. These included house officers, junior doctors, and senior professors, along with administrative staff and principals of medical schools who in the past had also been clinical practitioners. In order to persuade men to agree to giving interviews they were not only provided the requisite cover letter[1] detailing the objectives and benefits of the research but an appendix which included articles from academic journals and newspapers confirming empirical evidence of pervasive violence against women practitioners in Pakistan. Two male research assistants were part of my research team, and during the first meetings we held preliminary discussions with male practitioners to communicate the objective of the research and seek permission for interviews. At this stage some practitioners expressed confusion as to why I had chosen this topic for my research. They attempted to paternalistically and even condescendingly tell me why this was not a relevant or sensible subject to pursue. On being asked why, it was explained that though this was a 'hot women's empowerment topic'[2] to attract interest, it was also one which would shame my country and its people. Some male practitioners even concluded that I had received funding for this research from a foreign body[3]. This was precisely the reason why many male practitioners declined to be interviewed. They just had nothing to say about a subject which they felt was being exaggerated, irrelevant, and even 'made up' at the behest of inimical international agencies. Other men made very little eye contact with me during the introductory briefing. They were not comfortable talking or interacting with me, a woman, and instead only conversed with my male research assistants. This was to be expected in a segregated society like ours and was the reason why I had hired and trained male research assistants. With such men, if consent was given to hold interviews, only male researchers were assigned for the meetings in order to make the participant feel comfortable and get an honest response.

From discussions with male administrative heads,[4] I discovered that women practitioners are not recognized as equal or stable members of the health-force and consequently policies for their development and protection are not a priority. The professional attitude of men was that women should be grateful to be permitted to work and any complaints from their part related to lack of protection was a form of serious ingratitude, or worse, an exaggerated fabrication. In fact, most men in Pakistan feel that women either invite violence through their behaviour or sensationalize experiences of victimization to win unnecessary attention. In the main, I found that male leaders in Pakistan's healthcare setup conduct programmes and introduce policies with considerable gender blindness and that insensitive gender budgets exclude women from equitable employee benefits and development. The gender gap in compensation and remuneration for women practitioners contributes to their immigration abroad and even abandonment of the profession.

## Guilt and Blame-shifting

Men agreed that violence against women healthcare practitioners was a pervasive and critical problem in Pakistan. The moral dilemma for them was that it was necessary to remain within the patriarchal social order of witnessing violence and ignoring it. The recognition that violence was wrong and caused multiple levels of harm to the women they treated akin to daughters, sisters, and co-workers in a family setting was a source of guilt and embarrassment for many male participants. Thus, not only was it difficult for some men to accept that violence caused permanent and serious problems in women's lives, they found it easy to shift the blame on the women victims. A senior medical officer, with 27 years of work experience, who had worked in five public sector hospitals, accepted that violence existed but was extremely reluctant to discuss its causes. In his case, the excuse was a lack of time:

Yes, throughout my working life I have seen this problem [workplace violence against women practitioners]. It exists in all provinces, hospitals, and departments. What other questions do you have for me? This is a very long discussion that I would rather not have it as I have patients waiting. This is a hurtful topic for someone who has been in the profession as long as I have.

Informal social laws and community norms have not been challenged to discourage violence against women. Male practitioners discussed the difficulty and near impossibility of altering the social mechanisms which sustain violence against working women because they have existed for centuries and been passed down from generation to generation. It is also not just a case of traditions and family legacies but the dictates of and expiation by religious leaders which have taught men that violence is sanctioned by Islam. An assistant professor summarized the reality:

A woman is not a human but an object in our society. The traditional and religious belief is that she should be owned, controlled, and managed.

Male practitioners argued that it was not just women but also children and innocent groups that suffered due to the aggressive dictates of corrupt religious leaders who promoted corporal punishment and murder for heavenly rewards. Many participants argued that perhaps it was more important to address the sectarian and political problems of the region rather than issues of gender violence at the workplace. It appeared as though men wanted to push the issue of violence against women under the carpet by stressing that there were more important socio-political problems of relevance in Pakistan to focus on.

The interview prompts attempted to cover the consequences of violence such as physical and psychological damage along with professional barriers in role-delivery. Most participants concluded that it was the responsibility of women to alter the norms and policies to mitigate and eventually eradicate workplace violence. Men felt that their own gender would never be able to stop violence against women, as that would constitute a massive revolution against traditional community norms and also the abandonment of their 'manhood'. Participants feared that leading such a movement would cause them to be ridiculed or even ostracized in both professional and social circles. This was not a surprising admission as Pakistani men have not been known to be feminists or leaders in matters of gender equality. An assistant professor implied that women victims who are reluctant to report violence are guilty of sustaining violence through passivity and fear:

> Women practitioner victims are afraid to do anything about workplace violence. They absorb violence and aggression. This contributes to the belief [by health sector governance, co-workers, and the public] that no such problem exists. Fear

invites more violence. Women healthcare practitioners working in a man's world need to overcome their fears. If they face violence then they should report it without shame. What are they afraid of?

The difficulty in defining violence and whether an incident constitutes violence was discussed. Men added that accidental groping is often mistaken for sexual harassment and general verbal abuse as abuse targeted specifically against women. Women victims are commonly told by seniors and co-workers that they have misconstrued cases of aggression or abuse. The trivialization of events and reprimanding of victims is a common feature in the health sector which leaves women practitioners incapable of judging whether they have even faced violence, and dissuades them from reporting an incident. A young doctor admitted that there was great confusion in chaotic hospitals with regard to determining whether or not an act was one of violence:

Women doctors, especially the young ones, are regularly touched or grabbed. The problem is one does not know whether this happens accidentally, as a form of harassment, or out of fear. Recently a female surgeon from general surgery was very badly beaten up by a male relative of a patient who had expired. The incident was not considered violence against a woman practitioner but was defended as a natural reaction to the death of a family member. The general sympathy was with the perpetrator. Everyone insisted he had temporarily lost his senses due to grief and thus did not realize what he was doing. Of course, no one was willing to concede that he may have done this out of anger or because he knew that a woman would not be physically strong enough to defend herself.

Drawing upon the common theme of the *aam admi* (common man), many men blamed the male public for perpetrating violence in the public health sector. It was rationalized that an overwhelming majority of the patients and family attendants were poor and illiterate and they had regressive ideologies against women generally, and against working women in particular. Male practitioners described how a large majority of the ordinary male population was unable to compartmentalize women healthcare practitioners as being any different from their own suppressed and illiterate women at home. They theorized that most men could not accept that women healthcare practitioners were trained and qualified care providers, and consequently they vented dangerous emotions (such as anger, frustration, stress, hate desire, and fear) in their dealings with them. Their behaviour was described as being similar to how they treated their women relatives within the home.

In comparison, male practitioners were revered and respected as they were perceived as symbols of trust, relief, health recovery, and life by the illiterate male public. Notwithstanding their rural and illiterate belonging, it was revealed by male practitioners that given the tribal, feudal, and political connections with the *tehsils*, it was risky for women healthcare practitioners to resist and raise a voice against the male public. Many patients and family attendants were known to have traced the homes and families of women healthcare practitioners and revenge themselves for ill-treatment or disclosure of acts of violence through criminal activities such as threats, kidnapping, and even rape and homicide. A professor elaborated:

> I want to make it clear that male doctors rarely abuse women practitioners. Most violence is perpetrated by male patients and

family attendants. The public expects that a woman will always be a nurse, whereas a man will invariably be a doctor. So when this ideology is challenged and a woman doctor shows up, they are unable to accept it. Our society is deeply segregated because of religion and culture. This leaves many young men frustrated. Lack of contact with women consolidates the idea in the minds of most young men that women are nothing but sexual objects and many working women have been compared to prostitutes just because they leave home to earn an income. Workplace violence is a reality both for male and female medical professionals. This is because patients and family attendants are uncivil, illiterate, and desperate for better services. Nurses and LHWs, especially polio workers working in peripheral [villages] and distant areas, are most at risk. Emergency, medical, and paediatric departments are especially volatile. Most patients from rural areas do not consider women doctors to be competent and they refuse to accept their services. Also, they are known to ask for male doctors when a female doctor is on duty because they do not consider women to be competent doctors. We should remember that even if some patients are illiterate and from rural backgrounds, they still have connections. They usually have political backgrounds or links with political representatives from their rural areas. This encourages them to behave in abusive and violent ways.

I wanted to address the question of why violence seemed to be increasing notwithstanding the growing modernity and awareness in our region. Male participants provided an interesting perception of this in relation to the changing attitudes and behaviour of women healthcare practitioners. It was suggested that some Pakistani women had become extremely liberated through their exposure to social media, foreign cinema, and TV programmes (from India and the West), and the ease of making short and cheap international trips to modern Islamic countries and cities such as Dubai, Turkey, and Malaysia. Although from 'conservative and sensible' families, it was explained that the modern working woman encompasses many contradictory cultures which defies the traditional belief system. Women were found to converse at the workplace in the presence of myriad groups of conservative people and dress in a way that was not considered 'appropriate' or 'acceptable'. It was agreed that if all women practitioners adhered to a conservative dress code and attracted less attention, they would invite less aggression from the public. This was a curious suggestion on the part of male practitioners, who should be aware that women practitioners by virtue of their occupation have to interact with the public and command attention to optimally undertake their responsibilities. A senior registrar commented on the non-Islamic attire of certain women colleagues which made them vulnerable to greater violence:

> Have you seen how some of our women doctors and nurses dress? Those living in hostels and from upper-middle class families wear inappropriate or Western attire and this provokes our men. Wearing their hair loose and using makeup is another contributory factor. Men then believe it is acceptable to harass and catcall women practitioners as they are inviting such attention. Also, the knowledge that they [women healthcare practitioners] will not and cannot retaliate makes the men even more aggressive and persistent.

I wanted to learn what male reactions were after they had witnessed violence against women at the workplace. Recalling memories and describing incidents of violence against women colleagues was not a comfortable experience. Some were willing to share specific incidents, whereas others preferred to treat violence as an abstract phenomenon and victimized colleagues as illusory outsiders. They shared that violence against women was an acceptable practice and they chose to ignore it rather than raising their voices against it. Many concluded that to recognize it and make 'an issue of it' was equivalent to further victimizing the harassed. There was a sense of mutual disgrace and distress in acknowledging violence, so it was best to ignore it. A senior registrar described the standard male colleague blind-eye after having witnessed violence:

> I recall one incident. A junior colleague tried to molest a female doctor who had been transferred from a rural hospital to an urban hospital [a tertiary-care public sector hospital in Pakistan]. He didn't get caught because the girl feared that she might lose her job and reputation if she reported the incident. We [male colleagues] are aware of such men amongst us but because there is no known body at the workplace to which violence can be reported and it is culturally accepted to just ignore such things, we turn a blind eye. It is really the responsibility of women doctors and nurses to try to avoid such events.

## Administrative Legacies

I attempted to understand the opinions of male practitioners as to why significant concrete measures had not been undertaken by governing bodies to curtail violence against women and deter perpetrators. Many answered that it was a socio-professional norm in Pakistan to ignore violence against women, both within the home and at the workplace. In the health sector this was even more significant because health professionals are united in maintaining the image and respect both of the medical profession and the demigod image of the male doctor. The governing bodies of hospitals were in league to maintain the honour and dignity of the male-dominated health sector. It was said that public awareness and recognition of violence posed a threat to the reputation and status of male practitioners and would lead to undermining of male administrative control.

The shortage of budget allocations could never destroy the god-like image of male doctors but the recognition that some of them were perpetrators and sustainers of violence could contribute to the destruction of their unchallenged public authority and hegemony. This was also why men banded together unequivocally and mechanically to exonerate male perpetrators. Women practitioners were warned that they must remain silent about victimization, or else face the consequences of defamation and ostracization at the workplace. The medico-legal system in Pakistan was described as a legacy of the colonial times. It had major flaws such as the preservation of the Hudood, Qisas,[5] and Diyat[6] ordinances. The medico-legal officers in the public healthcare setup of Pakistan comprise men who are either ill-trained or altogether absent from the workplace. In addition, the association of forensic science and its coordination with legal bodies is politicized and corrupt. A senior professor admitted that violence against women is ignored to maintain the status of the profession and how women victims, who dare to report violence, are shamed and in turn accused in order to hide the seamy reality beneath.

Yes, violence is prevalent, but it is very embarrassing for medical professionals to admit this. After all the women we are working with are like our sisters and daughters. We do not want to disclose such embarrassing things and shame them. Doctors are worshipped in our society. After God, it is the male doctors to which the public turns in times of need. Any weaknesses in the profession are best brushed under the carpet for the sake of the public. A doctor once pushed a nurse so hard she slipped and cut her head. She was critically injured and lodged a complaint to the medical superintendent (MS). In response, the doctor counter-argued that the nurse had not been in her senses. He also got some colleagues to support him and complained to the MS that she was an addict who was regularly consuming drugs while on duty. The YDA also got involved in support of the doctor.

It was unbelievable that some men were not willing to recognize that suffering from violence has consequences not just on a woman's physical and mental health but also on her role delivery and therefore patient safety. I asked a senior principal about the macro problems of letting violence go unchecked, in terms of ignoring women practitioner safety and risking the recovery and mortality of patients. At this point in the interviews, contradictions became evident. It was suggested that the reality of extreme violence was exaggerated and only rare and mild incidents of violence occurred. However, the central theme of this discussion, which pressed home, was that governing and academic bodies have failed to educate and train doctors about the consequences of violence. Male doctors are particularly ignorant about the negative consequences of violence on the victim or on teamwork, error management, and patient safety. A senior professor in the field for 47 years complained about the lack of professionalism and personal ethics amongst women practitioners:

> I personally think that it [violence against women healthcare practitioners] is exaggerated; they [women healthcare practitioners] are safe. At most, they face verbal violence or harassment from patients and family attendants but that is to be expected in public hospitals. I agree that women may be bullied by male co-workers but that is because they cannot compete with men and neither can they do justice to senior administrative positions. If their services are not up to the standard, it is not because of victimization but because of their personal ethics and commitment. We cannot do anything about that.

Describing mild forms of violence[7] as inconsequential became a theme across the interviews. Participants argued that if violence was causing severe and lasting problems, women healthcare practitioners would have created a massive uproar or gone on permanent strikes by now. The power that women healthcare practitioners wielded was discussed in terms of both public hospitals and the Lady Health Programme not being able to function without them. Thus it was rationalized that their rebellion would secure punishment of perpetrators and also their security. A medical superintendent from Punjab recommended that women practitioners must resolve the problem of workplace violence themselves:

> Women healthcare practitioners really need to learn how to defend themselves. Stop blaming men. If it is such a problem, then they would have found a solution by now. The hospitals would after all close down in their absence. They have power.

This is proof that the violence that exists is only mild and inconsequential.

Male practitioners, like their female counterparts, strongly believed that the public hospital setting is a breeding ground for conflict and violence and that women bear the brunt of this predicament. It was also mentioned that the social costs and long hours of work are extremely difficult for women practitioners to bear and make them more vulnerable to multiple forms of violence. The description of public hospitals was confirmed as understaffed and under-resourced, causing frustration and anger, especially amongst helpless practitioners, patients, and family attendants struggling to save lives. Men insisted that hospitals should not be compared to other work organizations because of the high level of stress during care delivery and the possibility of having to communicate a fatal prognosis.

Women healthcare practitioners become easier targets for violence in turbulent hospital settings, where holding perpetrators accountable becomes impossible due to a lack of time and energy. Similarly, hysterical patients and family attendants find it easier to get away with taking out their aggravation on women practitioners. The stress of emergencies, mortality, disease, and public sector shortcomings has relegated violence against women to a trivial status. Men felt that their own gender became more aggressive at night-time and in male-dominated wards, where they perceived their strength to be greater. This is why departments such as surgery, medical, emergency wards, and night duties were identified as high-risks for women. A senior registrar described the physical environment and pressures of the trade which assisted in making violence against women practitioners commonplace:

> In the public hospital settings of Pakistan, and especially in emergency situations, there is great chaos and rush. Individual acts of violence and harassment become inconspicuous; perpetrators easily manage to get away with offences. If a woman practitioner is abused, slapped, or beaten, the most frequent response is: '*kuch nahi hua; chalta* hai' [Nothing much happened; let it pass!].

The failure of the current procedures for reporting workplace violence in the health sector was discussed. Reporting by women entails interaction with men who are not receptive to complaints and have little time or straightforward policies in place to deal with perpetrators and therefore the authorities resort to the customary option of shifting the blame to the victim. Existing laws and policies were examined with principals, heads of department, and senior administrators. All the officers were aware of workplace violence laws, the degrees of penalization and monitoring by governing bodies within the health sector, and the limitations of implementation. Serious cases of sexual assault, rape, and homicide that reached the courts and media led to no compensation for the victim or improvements in protection. It was concluded that until the health sector and national laws did not begin penalizing the male perpetrators and women remained afraid of reporting, violence would remain rampant. The problem of ineffective legal accountability was also discussed in the context of attitudes and cultural norms not supporting the implementation of laws. A senior head of department suggested that until operational strategies are not initiated by governing bodies to raise awareness about how to deal with violence, individual hospitals and leaders will not be able to help:

Currently, women victims are required to take their complaints to senior doctors or departmental and administrative heads. These are however usually men who are either the perpetrators themselves or who have been ignoring violence for many years. In such a situation, women rarely report and perpetrators have a free reign. Human resource departments in the hospitals are needed. You also need to have harassment seminars and workshops to understand what constitutes violence and the channels for reporting and penalization. One can only pray that people become aware of the seriousness of the problem and there is a change in their thought-processes; only in that way can we progress as a nation. The existing laws will make no difference until our mindset changes: if you bring in a law but women are too scared to seek help, then what is the purpose of making such meaningless laws?

An experienced MS recommended that maintaining strict segregation in hospitals was the only solution to controlling violence against women. He did not offer solutions on how violence could be mitigated for community workers like LHWs and for nurses who worked across all departments but it was interesting to identify that some men felt it was virtually impossible to eradicate men's violent attitudes towards women:

I don't think you can teach men to behave. The ones who are decent and non-violent come from their homes with such training. We cannot train or change men's nature; we have more important work to do here. It would be preferable to introduce strict discipline and segregation in public hospitals of Pakistan.

Each province's LHSs report to the provincial directors of the healthcare departments. Unsurprisingly, these directors have been and are currently all male. The director of the Punjab Healthcare Department was interviewed and although he admitted that as a man he could not understand exactly what it was like to face the problems of LHWs, he was able to describe some of the hurdles that had to be overcome to get the job done. The resilience and ability of the LHWs to withstand severe violence and opposition was described in a haughty and paternalistic manner. Overall it was agreed that violence against LHWs was common and prevalent but it existed due to the absence of structural support and community security for them. Two specific incidents with a religious leader and community men were quoted which showed how difficult it was for the LHWs to evade violence and also maintain their integrity in face of abuse:

It is not uncommon for LHWs to face physical aggression and force. They know that it is like this when they enter the profession. It is their choice. When they sense danger or threat, they mark a zero and move on to the next house. They are very brave women. Yes there are complaints to the centre. Recently the local maulana had a son and he refused to let us give the child polio drops. When questioned he swore on the Quran that no LHW had visited his home. In another incident an LHW was being badly harassed by two young brothers in the community. When the LHS went to speak to their parents, a huge ruckus resulted, with the father insisting that his *sharif* [pious] sons were being falsely maligned and that they considered the LHW to be their sister. What is the word of an LHW in presence of community men and local maulanas? We wish we had the money to send a guard with each LHW but that is not possible.

## Second-class Professionals

As interviews unfolded, the male participants admitted more and more freely that the violence faced by women healthcare practitioners was due to cultural ideologies and traditional practices. It was agreed that women are considered to be second-class citizens and the male practitioners felt this was a primary reason why women practitioners suffered sustained and cyclical violence at the workplace. The lives of working and non-working women remain interconnected and comparable. Unlike popular Western belief, working women do not achieve autonomy and social standing through their training and work participation. Violent behaviour follows women healthcare practitioners to their workplace and in the field as a consequence of the deeply inculcated dictates and lessons taught by family, religion, and culture. As women are treated akin to second-class citizens in the wider society, they are similarly treated as second-class professionals at the workplace.

The stratification of women not only makes violence against them acceptable by the public, but any effort to provide them with equal opportunities and security is opposed and rejected by socio-structural platforms. The recent women's protection bill that was proposed in Pakistan was discussed and also the reasons for why it was promptly and ruthlessly rejected by male stakeholders and prominent religious leaders. Burdened by inferior labels, the skill and output of women healthcare practitioners is repeatedly questioned through withdrawal of consent and abuse by patients and family attendants. An associate professor with 26 years of experience described the effects of primary socialization[8] on misogynistic attitudes across the community:

> The thing that keeps violence against women practitioners alive is the backward thinking of people that women are inferior to men. Even mothers train their sons to think in that way. The general mindset is that women as healthcare practitioners are weak and incompetent. Frequently we have patients or family attendants seeking to have their women doctor substituted by a male one.

There were many participants who admitted that they too believed that women healthcare practitioners were not comparable to their male counterparts. This was explained through their belief that women were not comparable to men in terms of knowledge and experience, training and specialization and also due to their shorter work hours, lack of private practice experience, and the burdens of marriage and childbearing. It was said that ward heads preferred to have fewer women doctors in their teams and that patients regularly asked for male doctors as an assurance of higher standards of healthcare delivery. A senior registrar described the link between perceptions of the professional inferiority of women colleagues and the violence they face:

> Women healthcare practitioners cannot be compared to men. They do not have foreign degrees or comparable training.

You will notice that women doctors and nurses are usually gossiping about each others' looks, home, and children at the workplace. We are all aware that the profession does not come first for them. That is why no one respects them and patients end up asking for male doctors when they are assigned women doctors. In the event that patients and family attendants are stuck with women doctors, they become more aggressive.

The injustice of violence being highlighted against women in the health sector specifically was discussed. Men felt that generally all women faced workplace violence in Pakistan and, because there were more women working in the health sector, the issue was being unnecessarily blown up and the health sector needlessly tainted. It was argued that as more women employees were found in the health sector in comparison to other sectors, and violence against women was intrinsic to the cultural norms of the society, it was inevitable that there would be a larger number of instances of violence there. The argument continued that patriarchal ideologies which justify gender-based violence at the workplace were consistent across Pakistan but were more evident in the health sector. One young doctor insisted it was not fair just to discuss violence in the health sector as it was a microcosm of wider community norms and a result of the failure to protect women across society, not just women healthcare practitioners:

Violence exists everywhere. Why just focus on the health sector? That's not fair. When you treat women as 'aadhi gawahi'[9], then what else can you expect? The protection of women must start from the homes and from general workplace laws. Once that is done, safety in hospital organizations will follow.

Male practitioners discussed how the class-belonging of victims and perpetrators played a significant role in violence. It was recommended that victims belonging to the lower classes need more structural support and that perpetrators from lower classes need more vigilance in the healthcare setup. Women healthcare practitioners from the low socio-economic strata, especially nurses, LHWs, and women doctors who have been transferred from different districts and are living without family encounter more workplace violence. Perpetrators know that punitive action or informal social controls will not be used against them when they target women belonging to a lower social class. Male practitioners insisted that the major onslaught of violence was perpetrated by men who: (1) belonged to lower middle class families, (2) have little intention of staying in the country, and (3) have fewer prospects for promotions and placement in significant administrative or leadership positions. A professor with several years of experience concluded:

> Women healthcare practitioners from the lower class face greater violence. Women who enter the profession from rural areas are even more vulnerable. They do not have the courage to report victimization and can easily be manipulated and scared by perpetrators.
>
> Additionally, it is the male lower class practitioners [such as junior doctors and house officers] who are more aggressive and violent. This is largely because such men are dissatisfied with their jobs, pay, and prospects for promotion. They [lower class male practitioners] are usually on the lookout for better jobs abroad and believe they are in Pakistan only for a temporary period. In this way, they [lower class male practitioners]

feel they have less to lose by committing violent acts at the workplace.

Although most of the participants were sympathetic and careful to differentiate themselves from perpetrators in their discussion about the causes of sustained violence against women healthcare practitioners, there were the occasional individuals who added rich information about male bias against women practitioners. When a few men became comfortable in the interview process, and also perhaps in the knowledge that the anonymous interviews could never be traced back to them or held against them, they shared significant male insights. It was mentioned that women healthcare practitioners were perhaps transgressing the social and Islamic order by interacting with non-relative males and that some of their dealings with men at the workplace were objectionable. Over-smart and verbally aggressive women healthcare practitioners were almost mentioned with disgust, as if the men had to bear a heavy cross in having to share a workplace and coordinate teamwork with them.

It was made clear that violence by male practitioners against hard-hitting and uncompromising women healthcare practitioners was inevitable in order to maintain discipline and control in the hospital setting. Many mentioned that when they encountered 'certain' women healthcare practitioners, they were immediately wary and on guard. Participants used a narrative style to describe 'other' male colleagues (perhaps meaning themselves but not wishing to admit it) who were forced to adopt measures of aggression and bullying to prevent women healthcare practitioners from exploiting them. An associate professor highlighted the attention-seeking and generally unmarried women healthcare practitioners who unnecessarily caused trouble for their male co-workers:

A woman's place is inherently her home. Any woman out of her home should be ready to face violent treatment. I have heard other male co-workers discussing that women practitioners' interaction and proximity to non-relative males and their ways of dressing are not appropriate. There is a stigma associated with female education and work participation even in the health sector. Angry men are almost killing two birds with one stone. Through abuse and violence, they can teach women a lesson for going against the cultural norms and also vent their anger on the inefficient care services, which are characteristic of public hospitals. Also, don't forget that some nurses and lady doctors just do not know their place. They make unnecessary trouble. They don't do their job on time and spend all their time complaining about aggression against them. Many have a habit of regularly bad-mouthing their male co-workers and supervisors. They are just seeking attention, and sometimes it is a part of a larger scheme to blame and take revenge themselves on a senior doctor or administrator.

The lack of public awareness about the status and respect which should be afforded to women healthcare practitioners was discussed. Men described how working women and women healthcare practitioners will always have a negative public image in Pakistan, regardless of their education, specialization, and ability. The importance of educating the general public about women's rights and the respect that should be accorded to working women, especially women healthcare practitioners was stressed. Similarly, the limited professions for women in Pakistan were acknowledged which further lower the status of women as workers overall. Apart from teaching, medicine was the only other profession considered suitable for women. There is difficulty in explaining this. Why, if medicine is an acceptable profession for women, are women healthcare practitioners still facing violence? This is because of the contradictions posed by segregation laws, where women healthcare practitioners are needed for female patients but in an organization in which their interaction cannot be restricted to just women. Their years in medical school, compulsory training rounds across departments, and choice of specialization in fields not just restricted to gynaecology keep them exposed to violence. Also, their vulnerability in needing to retain their professions and fears of reporting violence exposes them to perpetration. It was evident that men wanted their women relatives to become doctors but not nurses or LHWs. Also, to safeguard the honour and status of their women relatives, it was preferred that women remained restricted to either medical teaching or clinical practice for female patients alone. A male medical officer with six years of work experience suggested that women practitioners should be restricted to feminine specialties:

> It is not uncommon for us to hear of a nurse being slapped for petty things such as dropping a tray or something. You see nurses and LHWs go on strikes after getting beaten up or harassed but no one pays much attention to them. We encourage our female relatives to remain in specializations where female patients are dominant. Otherwise, we are asking for trouble. Paediatrics, gynaecology, and maternity are good fields for women.

Finally, men were asked about the ways in which women practitioners were spoken of or how they were referred to when men were alone together. Epithets are important indicators of what men actually feel and think about women healthcare practitioners. The frequent and familiar epithets used by male co-workers for women healthcare practitioners were discussed (listed in Box 1). Negative epithets such as 'jahil' and 'ganwaaar' were used for women who did not have the intelligence or the literacy to compete with male healthcare practitioners in the health sector, implying that they were second rate practitioners who would only create more 'musibat' or trouble for patients and co-workers. Acutely vulgar and offensive swear words were also used such as 'marasi' and 'kanjari', both of which alluded to immoral lower class women who sell either sexual favours or sing and dance for money. Finally, some women healthcare practitioners were also called 'marjan' which is akin to wishing a woman to hell for inappropriate and dishonourable behaviour. Even the honorific 'lady doctor' was used to mock women doctors in a disparaging sense. Male participants revealed that when men said 'lady doctor' they implied a female doctor who works in a man's world and is habituated to immoral behaviour and abuse by men, unlike a 'proper lady' who is sheltered within her own home and is not cognizant of the ways and mannerisms of men in the outside world. The insinuation by men is that women practitioners have been adulterated by their interaction with men and are no longer fit to be regarded as innocent or proper ladies.

8901234567890

## Box 1

Common negative epithet used for women healthcare practitioners.

| Local name | English translation | Common connotation |
|---|---|---|
| Lady doctor | Woman doctor | A woman doctor who cannot be considered a proper lady any longer because she has been interacting with non-relative males outside her home and has been exposed to indiscreet male behaviour. |
| Jahil | Ignorant | A woman who does not have the knowledge or intelligence to compete with men in the medical profession. |
| Gawaar | Illiterate | A woman who is either not trained at all or inadequately in medical sciences or health education; one who does not have the ability to learn about healthcare. |
| Musibat | Trouble | A woman who will create unnecessary problems during health administration and the treatment of patients. |
| Marasi | Lower caste singing ladies | A woman who is showing off or displaying herself, like women singers do for money. |
| Kanjari | Prostitute | A woman who sells her services for money; here care delivery is being likened to the sale of sexual services. |
| Marjani | A woman who belongs in hell | A woman who is destined for punishment in the afterlife for her work participation and interaction with non-relative males. |

# Conclusion

The revelation of hidden male voices in the health sector helps us to understand the helplessness of male practitioners in the face of long-standing traditions. Even men who do not endorse social ideologies of gender abuse are indirectly passive bystanders and witnesses of violence against women healthcare providers. Those who want to raise a voice for the protection of women co-workers are incontrovertibly ensnared by male brotherhoods and by the fear of community-shaming. The genesis and sustenance of violence against women also forms a part of structural legacies and informal organizational functioning. In these circumstances, the best means for men to deal with the reality of violence is by shifting blame on women victims and those members of the public who perceive women practitioners to be second-class professionals. The reflections of some men unambiguously confirmed an inherent misogynistic approach of blaming women for either exaggerating their experiences of violence or inviting violence upon themselves through incompetence or depravity.

Blaming illiterate, lower class, and unregulated populations functioning within the ambit of a non-punitive culture for men, was also an easy recourse for male practitioners which further enabled them to assume a mask of powerless innocence. Social improvements and organizational transformations are viewed as a secondary responsibility by men or worse as a threat to the status of the medical profession and the male practitioners in Pakistan.

# NOTES

1. Prospective participants were informed that the women working in the health sectors across the world faced high rates of workplace violence, and that the issue was more problematic in Pakistan given the cultural norms and religious misinterpretation prevalent there.

2. In Pakistan, the term 'women's empowerment' has become synonymous with the belief that foreign agencies and organizations fund women to rebel from their 'proper' place in society. Most initiatives for women's empowerment that are backed by international NGOs for small enterprise development, higher education, and family planning are usually frowned upon by male patriarchs and a majority of conservative families.

3. I found it somewhat unfair that certain male practitioners just assumed that I had received funding for this project, given that I had received no funding at all (local or foreign) and in fact had exhausted my personal resources for this research project. Also, I personally feel that workplace violence is not a 'hot' topic, fabricated by researchers and funded by the West to portray Pakistani culture as regressive, but a hard reality as proven in Chapter 1.

4. This included Medical Principals; Medical Supervisors; the Deputy Director of Health; and the President of the Pakistan Medical and Dental Council.

5. *Qisas* has its roots in retributive justice, or retaliation in kind, and is a part of the Islamic Penal Law. It has been misused by backward communities in terms of using women (forced marriage, murder, and rape) as retribution in the event that a family member of hers has wronged them in some way.

6. *Diyat* is an agreed financial compensation provided to the victims or relatives of victims.

7. Mild forms of violence include physical abuse (without permanent physical harm or damage), verbal abuse, sexual harassment, and professional bullying.

8. Primary socialization includes the lessons, values, and training individuals receive in their childhood and youth from their significant others (such as family, parents, siblings, and grandparents).

9. The Urdu term *aadhi gawahi* translates to mean half a witness. This refers to an interpretation of a Quranic verse in which the testimony of two women is equal to the testimony of one man.

# 7

# Women Practitioners Matter: Contesting Patriarchy for Care-Providers

One of the principal aims of this book is to generate a critical awareness of the urgent need to ensure the safety of women healthcare practitioners in Pakistan and devise effective mechanisms to achieve this. However, critical crises in virtually all spheres of national life have placed women's safety at the backseat in the policymaking agendas. These critical national problems include civilian attacks by the Taliban and ISIS, sectarian violence, political corruption, provincial tribal resurgence, border theft, economic stagnation, and frequent natural disasters. To direct policy initiatives for women's development, it will be crucial to raise awareness of the role women practitioners play in the overall patient safety and public health in Pakistan. Given the conservatism and patriarchal bent of Pakistani men, it is not surprising that the public at large have little awareness of the crucial role that women practitioners play for overall public wellbeing. Although one would expect that policies for women's protection in healthcare organizations across the world would be similar, it is important to consider that cultural and regional initiatives specific to Pakistan are needed to achieve zero tolerance of violence in its health sector.

## The Question of Women Practitioners' Rights

There has been a great deal of concentration on the rights of patients and the rights of practitioners in general, as outlined by the International Code of Medical Ethics of the World Medical Association (1995). There has, however, been little or no attempt to discuss the responsibilities of the public and male co-workers specifically toward women practitioners in Pakistan, and indeed in South Asia as a whole. This is critically important considering that women are perceived as the inferior gender and secondary professionals in patriarchal and socially regressive regions like Pakistan. Thus there is a need to identify the violation of socio-professional rights of women practitioners before we can attempt to draft policy initiatives for their workplace protection.

### Right to professional respect

Though the public and professionals are entitled to their own beliefs and morals, there is a benchmark for respect and dignity that must be afforded to women practitioners. Women practitioners have the right to gratitude from the public since the health needs of not just women, but men, the elderly, and children cannot be secured without the involvement of women in healthcare practice. Dignity and respect for women practitioners must be safeguarded by according them equal compensation and pay, opportunities for progress, and also participation in governance (Murphy & Graff 2006; Sasso et al. 2011).

Rather than being considered inferior, they should be the recipients of the highest esteem for undertaking multiple roles in the homes and at the workplace. Respect is due, not just to women who choose to remain in the confines of their home, but to women who choose to work outside the home and in non-feminized specializations. Out of home work participation and interaction with non-blood male relatives must not be considered an immoral practice for professionally trained women practitioners who are providing the public with health recovery.

Women practitioners in Muslim countries have the right to be accorded the same eminence afforded to the women companions of the Prophet Muhammad (PBUH) (Ansari & Nadvi 2001). Historical facts from the Prophet's era confirm that women healthcare providers have a right to social mobility, equal compensation, honorary situation of their clinics in the vicinity of mosques, and general community respect for providing care to even non-blood male relatives.

## Right to patient consent and trust

Women practitioners require patient consent and trust to be able to deliver optimal services and fulfil their professional responsibilities (Sheppard et al. 2004, Thom et al. 2004). Large sections of the public refuse to receive treatment and services from women practitioners because they nurture an erroneous belief that they are inferior to male practitioners. The public also resists women practitioner care and counsel when it extends to family planning, maternal health, and child immunization given the common misconception that harmful Western care practices are being administered. This compromises the level of job satisfaction, sense of accomplishment, and extent of involvement in role delivery for women practitioners which is a slap in the face for their years of study and service.

Regardless of the class, religion, sect, or ethnicity of the woman practitioner, she has a right to being accorded trust, gratitude, and respect by her clients. If practitioners are liable to display cultural awareness, then patients and male co-workers must also be made to equally respect the cultural differences of women practitioners. Women practitioners have the right to be trusted and appreciated for their important role in safeguarding maternal and child health. The public has an obligation to receive the care and counsel of women practitioners and follow their direction too if they are to achieve health standards. They not only have the right to serve in feminized professions (such as obstetrics and gynaecology, midwifery, community health, and nursing), but also in all other healthcare specializations deemed 'masculine'.

### Right to co-worker support

Women practitioners should have equal rights to expect support and prospects of development from the currently existing male hierarchies of supervisors and administration. Women practitioners must also be granted equal respect and status as integral team members of the health workforce (Hall 2005; Weller et al. 2011). Professional bullying, sidelining, resort to sexual and gendered innuendos, or the humiliation of women practitioners is a violation of professional rights. Women practitioners deserve to be spoken to, coordinated with, and consulted by their co-workers and senior colleagues. Optimal co-worker support will also ensure maximum teamwork productivity and patient safety.

There is a need to develop unity and solidarity through the mobilization of a strong united union of women practitioners (Lincoln & Guillot 2004). Leading women practitioners and administrators in Pakistan have admitted that they would benefit from each other's support and unity to overturn injustices and inequalities (Rizvi Jafree et al. 2015). Women practitioners in the past have had success in looking within their minority community and fighting for their rights rather than relying solely on the assistance of the male majority (Brown et al. 2006; Ross-Kerr et al. 2003). An organization linking doctors, nurses, and healthcare teams would create mutual respect, goal integration, adaptability, and complementary care delivery in the sphere of healthcare.

## Right to breach of confidentiality when women patients are at risk

Basic professional medical laws require practitioners to ensure the interests and welfare of a patient (Hyman et al. 1995). Treating a woman victim of domestic violence as a regular patient and sending her back to her perpetrator without reporting the crime places the female patient at risk of cyclical violence. Although doctors follow a code of patient confidentiality, women practitioners in Pakistan must be legally entitled to share confidential information about female patients at risk of domestic violence and neglect at the hands of husband and family, and also violence and neglect at the hands of male practitioners at the workplace. Women practitioners have greater knowledge about violence against women within homes and at the hospital; they must be given legal rights and protection to share confidential information concerning both women patients in the hospital and women clients in the community.

## Right to report errors in a non-punitive culture

Magnet hospitals in developing countries have already established that regular and standardized reporting of errors is one of the most important administrative tools to safeguard patient safety (Armstrong et al. 2009). However, error-sharing is only successful in work organizations which do not blame the individual for reporting. Women practitioners have the right to report errors without being blamed for doing so or facing retribution from co-workers and patients. Blaming women practitioners for errors in male-dominated work teams and patriarchal societies (Hashemi et al. 2012), promotes further errors and adverse events at the workplace.

In addition, a blame-culture encourages women practitioners to adopt coping strategies of providing a lower level of care and reducing interaction with patients and co-workers at the workplace. Instructors must be held accountable for instructing practitioners about types of violence, types of errors, and also encouraging a culture of error-reporting (Barnsteiner 2011). Withdrawal of optimal services to prevent punitive reactions places patients at risk and also reduces women practitioners' job satisfaction. The reporting of errors enables optimal role-delivery by practitioners and patient safety should become the primary professional objectives. Women practitioners must have the right to report errors with autonomy, dignity, and job security, and their decisions must be respected by their supervisors and teams.

## Right to a learning-based culture

Male-dominated hierarchies in Pakistan's health sector have reserved whatever modest training they have for the men, depriving women practitioners of skill-development resources. Similar patterns related to training have been found in the West (Bewley 1996; Keenan & Kennedy 2003) and in Pakistan regarding unequal treatment of women practitioners (Ariff et al. 2010; Butt 2006; Omer et al. 2008). During clinical training, women practitioners are sidelined and penalized for asking questions given the accepted culture of women being expected to remain silent and accommodating in line with traditional teaching and instructional styles. A non-learning and non-questioning culture such as this negates the development of women practitioners and their development of innovative care solutions to facilitate the overall public health outcomes of Pakistan. Learning-based training is a fundamental determinant for the absorption of knowledge through a culture of questioning and thereby enhancement of competence. Women practitioners have the right to learning-based training both in educational institutions and during workplace instruction. Women practitioners also have the right not to be castigated by instructors for asking questions and not face reprimands for seeking learning and process oriented trainers.

## Right to report violence

Women practitioners and patients currently do not have easily accessible and unbiased bodies to which they can report acts of violence (D'Oliveira et al. 2002; Somani 2012). Women have the right to well-being, dignity, and safety, without which they cannot be expected to adequately and efficiently fulfil their roles at the workplace or within their homes. Women practitioners have the right to easily accessible, visible, and anonymous bodies to report acts of violence. They have the right to be heard and represented without retribution and plead their cases before able institutions, or a state court, to obtain redressal and protection. A woman practitioner who reports violence against herself or a female patient has the right to the respect and support of governing bodies and co-workers, as such disclosure helps to deter perpetrators in the future and secure the recovery of victims. Women practitioners have the right to medical attention, counselling, and leave from work after facing abuse.

## Right to withdrawal of services

Withdrawal of services is permitted when the care provider is at risk of physical and mental harm, and is unable to secure the patients' well-being (Ogbimi & Adebamowo 2006). Women practitioners should have the right to withdraw healthcare services when they fear for their safety or when their role delivery has been violated by patients, family attendants, or co-workers. The patients must be communicated this information and be provided with a replacement to fulfil the healthcare provision in the event of a practitioner withdrawing services.

Notwithstanding the complexity of balancing this equation in unstable and inadequate settings, women practitioners have the right, even when they are the only providers available, to first save themselves from violence and harm.

## Policy Direction

In the course of my research, I have been able to interact with women practitioners at their place of work, analyse the existing condition of the health sector, and also use information from an extended literature review to recommend policy interventions which would help to contextually secure safety at the workplace for women practitioners in Pakistan.

### Regular and standardized appraisal and monitoring

Surveys should be regularly conducted in every public hospital and BHU of Pakistan to pinpoint types of violent incidents, types of perpetrators, and the impact on victims. Longitudinal and consistent assessment by third party agencies, and not the government, would help monitor and develop appropriate policies over the long run to gradually eliminate workplace violence from the health sector. Official and standardized records to monitor the prevalence, frequency, and changes in the form of workplace violence faced by women practitioners would ensure that policy directives are put in place, improved, and appraised for efficacy.

## Gender solidarity and union mobilization

Leading women health administrators and senior practitioners must take the lead in establishing an effective union. Separate unions for women nurses, doctors, and LHWs have not been successful in having a lasting impact or in bringing about improvements in safety and benefits. The primary objective of a women practitioner union of Pakistan should be the eradication of violence and harassment against females in the healthcare sector. Issues relating to gender equality, compensation (minimum working hours and overtime pay), employee benefits, and maternal benefits should follow. The union can gain strength by encouraging compulsory membership and attendance at regular meetings to ensure that it serves as a platform for communication, social support, and debriefing. One of the most common tools used by unions is in the form of strikes and protests. The threat of revoking services in work spaces which cannot survive without woman practitioners can help generate pressure to guarantee safety measures against violence, and also secure development in other areas such as training and governance participation. Apart from strikes, union leaders function as representatives to liaise with the health administration to secure workplace safety and development for women practitioners in a non-disruptive manner.

## Budget allocations for safety, staffing, and resources

There is a great need to increase budget allocations to target gender-based violence in the health sector. Corruption in the healthcare sector and embezzlement of government funds has already been documented, with public health units and hospitals in Pakistan described as being devoid of basic and life-saving medicines and medical equipment (Pappas et al. 2009). According to the 2010 National Finance Commission, provinces have the jurisdiction to allocate additional fiscal resources to support critical areas. This power must be utilized by the provincial governments through increasing budget allocations to set up committees and recruit specialized staff to monitor and mitigate violence. Budget allocations are also required to recruit a larger number of women practitioners[1] and to procure the necessary medicines, medical resources, and vital medical equipment, as a shortage of these contribute substantially to violence against women practitioners. When staffing and resources in public hospitals and healthcare service centres are adequate there will be less violence against women practitioners and a marked improvement in care plans.

## Violence and harassment reporting office

The organized monitoring and accountability of workplace violence in the health sector of Pakistan requires the presence of permanent professional teams with visible office space in each hospital and district health office across Pakistan,[2] possibly called the Violence and Harassment Reporting Office (VHRO). Teams at the district health office, responsible for LHWs, must regularly visit each BHU, thereby providing ease of access to every LHW and LHS. Each VHRO should have women professionals, including a medico-legal officer, forensics officer, and clinical psychologist. The governance and reporting of the VHRO should be to a third party ministry such as the law or women's ministry, with integral joint reporting to an international agency such as CEDAW or UN Women.

Special coordination must be ensured across hospitals, district health centres, and police stations so that the VHRO can be accessed also by women patients. Awareness about the services needs to be widely disseminated to the public and especially amongst housewives in rural areas, along with the information that shelters will be provided for women and their dependent children once the cases have been reported and filed. It is recommended that increased security and immediate visible deterrence for perpetrators of violence against women practitioners can be achieved through the installation of Violence Protection Guards (VPG) at public hospitals. These VPGs must also be stationed at district health centres and accompany LHWs on random but frequent visits to homes. This will also create more jobs in the health sector and lead to long-term economic benefits in terms of decreasing national unemployment.

## Learning-based training and cultural competency

The professional development of woman practitioner and the consequent impact on patient safety are suffering due to inadequate training and education provided by the healthcare administration. Adequate training and the cultural competence of women practitioners can prevent violence against them in Pakistan. It is recommended that regulatory bodies responsible for the training and curriculum development of practitioners in Pakistan, including the Pakistan Medical and Dental Council (PMDC), the Pakistan Nursing Council (PNC), and the National Programme for Family Planning and Primary Health Care (NP-FP&PHC), work to: (1) update the medical curriculum of the women practitioner training institutes, (2) provide equal opportunities for women practitioners for on-the-job training in medical advances, (3) provide training in violence, error-reporting, and cultural competence, and (4) invest in quality teachers and teaching resources in training institutes.

## Error-reporting culture and systems

It is important to invest time and resources to train healthcare employees to adopt a more progressive, non-blame culture and encourage an error-reporting culture amongst co-workers before introducing more formal and expensive error-tracking systems.[3] This may be done through regular training sessions and by holding collective group seminar sessions for doctors, physicians, and nurses.[4] The code of ethics for healthcare workers in Pakistan is theoretically drafted and communicated by PMDC and PNC. Until laws are altered, in order to immediately improve error-reporting, it is also recommended that: (1) anonymous error-reporting boxes are placed across all wards, and (2) the PMDC and PNC hold monthly court sessions to protect whistle-blowers who are being penalized for reporting errors. An improvement in the error-reporting culture can ensure optimal care delivery by practitioners, prevention of adverse events, lower cost for the health institutions, and more efficient channelization of budgets and resources (Leape 2002).

## Additions to medical jurisprudence

Women practitioners have front line experience of the regional problems that they face. These include domestic violence, neglect of maternal health, lack of decision-making power over child immunization and child health, and violence at the hands of medical practitioners. It is recommended that women practitioners be held legally accountable by state courts of law to report the violence and neglect suffered silently by female patients. Strict clauses guiding medical jurisprudence should be introduced that concern reporting of violence against female patients. Women practitioners who fail to ensure holistic protection for women patients and clients in the name of confidentiality should be made to face the appropriate consequences.

If women practitioners begin reporting their knowledge of violence against silent women patients, the victims will need support through shelters. There is a need for extended and intensive coordination and funding by the government for the survival and protection of women victims. Manuals should be designed to communicate information across communities in Pakistan about the importance of reporting violence, the means to do so, and the provision for assistance. Special manuals and training must be provided to women practitioners on how to deal with victims of domestic violence and female patients facing violence at hospitals.

If domestic violence and intimate partner violence is to be accurately estimated and eliminated in Pakistan, there needs to be authorized mandatory routine screening across its public sector hospitals and BHUs. The American Medical Association initiated universal screening for domestic violence several years ago, with a successful increase of 30 per cent in reportage.

## Debarring family attendants

A number of family attendants are present with patients in public sector hospitals and this is a source of great strain and anxiety for women practitioners. Not only does the presence of so many attendants in the work areas creates a dearth of physical space and raises noise levels, but it also compromises care delivery of the practitioner and her exclusive concentration on the patient. More importantly, family attendants have been unanimously described as being more abusive, aggressive, and violent against women practitioners than any other type of perpetrator. It is recommended that laws are instituted to exclude multiple family attendants in Pakistan's public hospitals, with only a single family attendant allowed during limited visiting hours in the day. This would ensure women practitioner safety and also optimize their role delivery, ultimately leading to increased patient safety.

## Social status of women practitioners

Socio-cultural norms, traditional patriarchal beliefs, and religious misinterpretation continue to guide Pakistani society toward the dehumanization and victimization of women practitioners. The social status and identity of women healthcare practitioners and other working women can be greatly improved through the following reforms, though there is a need for strategic harmony and impact evaluations to determine which non-permanent interventions need to be continued:

(1) Religious leaders must advocate the importance of women practitioners in Islam through mediums such as the Friday and Eid congregational sermons, TV lectures, radio broadcasts, and pamphlets.

(2) Media campaigns through news channels, cinema, TV dramas, and advertisements are needed to change the mindset of the public about the status of women healthcare practitioners and their role in the public well-being and health recovery.

(3) Political parties need to campaign on the issue of the importance of women workers for the achievement of national goals and development.

(4) The educational system, from primary to graduate levels, must formally include curricula and training relating to the status and treatment of women workers. Peer education and awareness workshops should be regularly conducted by men and women practitioners and health administrators.

(5) There must be complete eradication of unskilled jobs for nurses, such as changing and cleaning patients. These responsibilities should be devolved to unskilled male ward boys and female cleaners (or maids) already employed in public sector hospitals.

(6) The nurses and LHW practitioners must be provided with professional [5] and technical training to operate ultrasound machines, conduct minor surgical procedures, and reading of lab reports.

(7) The uniforms of medical professionals in the hospitals and community should be standardized to reduce status differentiation and professional tribalism.

There is no harm in nurses and LHWs all wearing doctors' coats.

## Public prosecution of perpetrators

The provincial health commissioners currently have the jurisdiction to manage the medical courts of law in legal cases, including cases concerning violence and harassment.[6] It is recommended that an independent body, other than the health commission, should be responsible for the investigation of violence and punitive action against perpetrators. The health commissions, in conjunction with an independent body, must actively work to withdraw licences of practitioner perpetrators of violence, investigate the workings of councils such as the PMDC and PNC, and develop a system to track, monitor, and mitigate violence and errors in the public healthcare sector. In addition, licences of quack practitioners or those repeatedly responsible for practicing medical negligence need to be revoked.

## Participation of women practitioners in governance

There is a need for an increase in the gender-equal quotas for women representation in governing positions in the health sector. The posting of women healthcare practitioners to major posts at the hospital and as district officers would improve the reporting of and accountability for violence and also improve the safety and equity standards for women patients.[7] The foundations of quality care will also be improved by supplanting the male medical professional hierarchy and granting women practitioners autonomy in devising care plans.

## Workplace violence bill for women

Notwithstanding the existence of ministerial bodies with state representation, such as the Ministry of Women's Development; the Committee on the Elimination of All Forms of Violence; and the Ministry of Social Welfare and Special Education, no progressive and comprehensive laws exist in Pakistan to specifically protect women medical practitioners. There is an urgent need to remove the constraints in reporting workplace violence through improvement in legal and judicial laws. It is recommended that strong women practitioner unions, donor groups, and women development groups[8] band together to lobby in political circles and generate civilian pressure for the legal protection of women healthcare practitioners.

A labour bill of rights specifically for the protection of women medical practitioners is recommended with features addressing: (1) violence, harassment, and safety, and (2) other employee standards such as maternal benefits, minimum work hours, equal compensation, and promotions. Specific attention must be given to the: (1) penalization of health practitioners when they are found to be perpetrators of violence, (2) protection of women practitioners against wrongful claims of impropriety and malpractice by the public and co-workers, and (3) enforcement of a protection programme for women victims and witnesses who have reported cases of violence.

## Global initiatives

An important thing to note is that no international treaty has been signed to prohibit violence against women healthcare practitioners.[9] At the United Nations (UN), three Security Council Resolutions (1325, 1820, and 1888) have been signed which address violence against women in armed conflict and women's participation in establishing peace (Raab 2012). A collective and global initiative such as a UN resolution for the protection of women care-providers (including nurses, community workers or field practitioners, doctors, dentists, and paramedical staff) would help to improve the status and administrative measures to protect women practitioners across individual nations. Such a treaty would also ensure that international monitoring bodies could work more effectively as third parties to help develop solutions and target failures in the protection of women practitioners.

# Conclusion

This chapter has outlined the important professional rights that should accrue to women practitioners in Pakistan. It may be that, with relevant modifications, these professional rights have some practical worth for other working women in Pakistan also. This book has highlighted how workplace violence in Pakistan's health sector is a salient and far-reaching public health and human rights concern. The perceptions and narrative accounts of both women victims and male co-workers have enabled us to comprehend the causes, precipitators, and opportunities for the mitigation of workplace violence against women healthcare practitioners. The legacy and normalization of violence against women in South Asia from a socio-cultural, structural, and religious angle have each been explored. At a micro-level it has been demonstrated that the ramifications for perpetrators are so meagre that the cycle of violence becomes entrenched. It is therefore essential to organize and mobilize on a massive scale the primary and secondary stakeholders such as health governance bodies, the political, religious, legal authorities, the public at large, and the media to play central roles in transforming social identities and the professional status of women practitioners as equal providers and not secondary professionals in the healthcare workforce.

# References

Ansari, Saeed, and Syed Suleman Nadvi (2001): *Women Companions of the Holy Prophet and their Sacred Lives* (Bombay, India, Bilal Books).

Ariff, Shabina, et al. (2010): 'Evaluation of health workforce competence in maternal and neonatal issues in public health sector of Pakistan: An assessment of their training needs', *BMC Health Services Research*, 10 (1): 319.

Armstrong, Kevin, Heather Laschinger, and Carol Wong (2009): 'Workplace empowerment and magnet hospital characteristics as predictors of patient safety climate', *Journal of nursing care quality*, 24 (1): 55–62.

Barnsteiner, Jane (2011): 'Teaching the culture of safety', *The Online Journal of Issues in Nursing:* 16 (3).

Bewley, Beulah R. (1996): 'Women Doctors: A Review', *Journal of the Royal Society of Medicine*, 89 (6): 359.

Brown, Gary D., et al. (2006): 'The 1999 Irish nurses' strike:

Nursing versions of the strike and self-identity in a general hospital', *Journal of Advanced Nursing*, 56 (2): 200–8.

Butt, Manzoor A. (2006): 'Skilled health workers: A solution to primary health problems in Pakistan', *Middle East J. Family Med*, 4: 1–4.

d'Oliveira, Ana Flávia Pires Lucas, Simone Grilo Diniz, and Lilia Blima Schreiber (2002): 'Violence against women in healthcare institutions: an emerging problem', *Lancet*, 359 (9318): 1681–85.

Hall, Pippa (2005): 'Interprofessional teamwork: Professional cultures as barriers', *Journal of Interprofessional Care*, 19 (sup1): 188–96.

Hashemi, Fatemeh, Nasrabadi, et al. (2012): 'Factors associated with reporting nursing errors in Iran: A qualitative study', *BMC Nursing*, 11 (1), 20.

Hyman, Ariella, Dean Schillinger, and Bernard Lo (1995): 'Laws mandating reporting of domestic violence: Do they promote patient well-being?', *Jama*, 273 (22): 1781–7.

Keenan, Patricia, and John F. Kennedy (2003): 'The nursing workforce shortage: Causes, consequences, proposed solutions', *Issue Brief (Commonwealth Fund)*, 619: 1–8.

Leape, Lucian L (2002): 'Reporting of adverse events', *New England Journal of Medicine*, 347 (20): 1633.

Lincoln, James R., and Didier Guillot (2004): 'Durkheim and organizational culture', Institute for Research on Labor and Employment (IRLE) Working Paper, Berkeley.

Murphy, Evelyn, and E.J. Graff (2006): *Getting Even: Why Women Don't Get Paid Like Men—and what to do about it* (New York, Touchstone).

Ogbimi, Roseline I., and Clement A. Adebamowo (2006): 'Questionnaire survey of working relationships between nurses and doctors in University Teaching Hospitals in Southern Nigeria', *BMC Nursing*, 5 (1): 2.

Omer, Khalid, et al. (2008): 'Evidence-based training of frontline health workers for door-to-door health promotion: Pilot randomized controlled cluster trial with Lady Health Workers in Sindh Province, Pakistan', *Patient Education and Counseling,* 72 (2): 178–85.

Pappas, Gregory, et al. (2009): 'Governance and Health Sector Development: A case study of Pakistan', *Internet J. World Health Societal Politics:* 7, 1.

Raab, Michaela (2012): 'Ending Violence against Women: A Guide for Oxfam Staff', Oxfam International, available at http://www. oxfam. org/sites/www.oxfam.org/files/ending-violence-against-women-oxfam-guide-nov2012. pdf (last checked by the author 23 June 2015).

Rizvi, Jafree, et al. (2015): 'Gender segregation as a benefit: A qualitative study from Pakistan', *Journal of Nursing Management,* 23 (8): 983–93.

Ross-Kerr, Janet C. et al. (2003): 'Emergence of nursing unions as a social force in Canada', *Canadian Nursing: Issues and Perspectives*: 280–300.

Sasso, Anthony T. Lo, et al. (2011): 'The $16,819 pay gap for newly trained physicians: The unexplained trend of men earning more than women', *Health Affairs,* 30 (2): 193–201.

Sheppard, Vanessa B., et al. (2004), 'Providing health care to low-income women: A matter of trust', *Family Practice,* 21 (5): 484–91.

Somani, Rozina Karim (2012): 'Workplace violence towards nurses: A reality from the Pakistani context', *Journal of Nursing Education and Practice,* 2 (3):148.

Thom, David H., et al. (2004): 'Measuring patients' trust in physicians when assessing quality of care', *Health Affairs,* 23 (4): 124–32.

Weller, Jennifer M., Mark Barrow, and Sue Gasquoine (2011):

'Interprofessional collaboration among junior doctors and nurses in the hospital setting', *Medical Education*, 45 (5): 478–87.

World Medical Association (ed.), (1995): *The International Code of Medical Ethics, Journal of Forum for Medical Ethics Society*, (3): 78.

# NOTES

1. The ratio of nurse-to-doctor and the ratio of women doctor-to-male doctor is critically disproportionate. Much of the violence faced by women practitioners is due to their understaffing and weak representation. The share of budget allocation for the educating, training, and hiring of women practitioners needs to be increased. Also, adequate remuneration needs to be allocated for the retention of woman practitioners within the public sector; in order not to lose them to the private sector or to immigration options (as developed countries hiring women practitioners from Pakistan have better safety standards and compensation).

2. Many of the medico-legal centres in public sector hospitals of the country are non-functional. Most of the medico-legal officers that do exist are males who are incapable of providing support to women victims of violence.

3. The ideal solution to reducing errors in healthcare services is to launch an error-tracking system with complete monitoring and accountability for non-reporting. Such systems are available and can be adopted from successfully performing hospitals of developed nations. Installing error-tracking systems can also create service sector jobs in the healthcare sector and raise national employment. However, such systems are expensive to install and maintain, especially for developing nations like Pakistan.

4. Researchers like Hofstede (1980) have theorized that altering the culture of an organization is easier than altering the culture of an entire nation; especially if remuneration, promotions, and bonuses are ultimately linked to increased error-reporting and the support of a non-blame culture.

5. In context of the problem of professional advancement, low professional status and negative identity for nurses and LHWs, it is recommended that the nurses and LHWs be propped with relevant and overtly

manifest props and facilities in the hospitals and the BHUs. These physical reinforcements, as suggested by actor network theory, would help to emphasize the importance of practitioner job and also alter public opinion about their status. For example, separate offices, front-desk enclosures in wards, practitioner kits (nurse trays or LHW medical box), and assistant ward-boys for nurses would help to define superior status.

6. The Punjab Healthcare Commission (PHC) is the official government regulatory body that has the authority to improve the quality of healthcare service provision and clinical governance in the province of Punjab. However, I found during my research that practitioners interviewed from this region repeatedly suggested that there is grave medical negligence and ethical violations in the healthcare sector of Pakistan, which goes unnoticed by the PHC. In effect, PHC was deemed as useless or dishonest in dealing with fraudulent and violent practitioners.

7. Public sector hospitals are allocating practitioners and resources according to patient demographics and VIP status. This is a violation of equity in healthcare services. Monitoring and accountability bodies within the public healthcare organizations must be established to oversee equitable distribution of medical and nursing care services and medical resources to all patients. In addition, patients from low income backgrounds, especially women patients and those with language and knowledge barriers, must be protected by third party monitoring agents (employed by the healthcare sector and allocated to each hospital) to ensure patient consent and safety at all times.

8. Women development groups, such as Edhi; Madadgaar; United Nations Human Rights Commission of Pakistan (UNHRCP); Aurat Foundation; Shirkat Gah; War Against Rape; and Acids Survivor Foundation Pakistan.

9. Some of the existing treaties are: The 1979 Convention on the Elimination of All Forms of Discrimination against Women; The 1993 African Union Protocol to the African Charter on Human and People's Rights on the Rights of Women in Africa; The 1994 Inter-American Convention on the Prevention, Punishment, and Eradication of VAW; The 2011 Council of Europe Convention on preventing and combating violence against women and domestic violence.

# Bibliography

Abbas, Hassan (2014): *The Taliban Revival: Violence and Extremism on the Pakistan-Afghanistan Frontier* (New Haven: Yale University Press).

Aftab, Tahera (2007): *Inscribing South Asian Muslim Women: An Annotated Bibliography & Research Guide* (Netherlands, Brill).

Ahmed, A. S. (Ed.). (1990): *Pakistan: The Social Sciences' Perspective* (Pakistan: Oxford University Press).

Akram, M., & Khan, F. J. (2007): *Health Care Services and Government Spending in Pakistan (No. 22184)* (East Asian Bureau of Economic Research, Pakistan Institute of Development Economics).

Ali, A. A. (2000): *The Emergence of Feminism among Indian Muslim Women, 1920–1947* (Pakistan: Oxford University Press).

Ansari, Saeed, Abdussalam Nadvi, and Syed Suleman Nadvi (2001): *Women Companions of the Holy Prophet and their Sacred Lives* (India: Bilal Books).

Ayub, R., & Siddiqui, S. (2013): *Community Health Workers of Pakistan and their Attrition* (Lulu.com).

Ayub, Romana, and Saad Siddiqui (2013): *Community Health Workers of Pakistan and their Attrition* (North Carolina, USA, Lulu Press).

Bhutta, Z. A. (Ed.). (2004): *Maternal and Child Health in Pakistan: Challenges and Opportunities* (USA: Oxford University Press).

Bodley, Ronald Victor Courtenay (1970): *The Messenger: The Life of Muhammad* (California: Greenwood Press Rpt).

Bowie, V., Fisher, B. S., & Cooper, C. (Eds.). (2012): *Workplace Violence* (USA: Routledge).

Chappell, Duncan, and Vittorio Di Martino (2006): *Violence at Work* (Geneva, International Labour Organization).

Chew, Dolores (2002): *'The Search for Kathleen McNally and Other Chimerical Women: Colonial and Post-Colonial Gender Representations of Eurasians', Translating Desire: The Politics and Gender of Culture in India* (New Delhi: Katha).

Closser, S. (2010): *Chasing Polio in Pakistan: Why the World's Largest Public Health Initiative may Fail* (Tennessee: Vanderbilt University Press).

Dall, Caroline Wells Healey (1888): *The Life of Dr. Anandabai Joshee: A Kinswoman of the Pundita Ramabai* (Boston: Roberts Brothers).

De Beauvoir, S. (2014): *The Second Sex* (Great Britain: Random House).

Delphy, C. (2016): *Close to Home: A Materialist Analysis of Women's Oppression* (United States: Verso Books).

DeSouza, Eros R., and Joseph Solberg (2003*): 'Incidence and Dimensions of Sexual Harassment across Cultures', in Academic and Workplace Sexual Harassment: A Handbook of Cultural, Social Science, Management, and Legal Perspectives* (USA: Praeger Publishers).

Dhammika, Shravasti (1993): *The Edicts of King Asoka*, (Buddhist Publication Society).

Diener, Edward and Rick Crandall (1978): *Ethics in Social and Behavioral Research* (Chicago: University of Chicago Press).

Ehrenreich, Barbara (2010): *Witches, Midwives, and Nurses: A History of Women Healers* (City University of New York: Feminist Press).

Engineer, A. A. (2001): *Islam, Women, and Gender Justice*, in *What Men Owe to Women: Men's Voices from World Religions* (United States: SUNY Press).

Friedlander, Peter (2009): *'Buddhism and Politics'*, in *Routledge Handbook of Religion and Politics*, ed. Jeffrey Haynes (New York: Routledge).

García-Moreno, C., & Riecher-Rössler, A. (2013): *Violence against Women and Mental Health*, in *Violence against Women and Mental Health* (Germany: Karger Publishers).

Ghadanfar, Mahmood Ahmad (2001): *Great Women of Islam* (Riyadh, Saudi Arabia: Darussalam Publishers).

Giddens, Anthony (1979): *Central Problems in Social Theory: Action, Structure, and Contradiction in Social Analysis* (Berkeley: University of California Press).

Glubb, John Bagot (1963): *The Great Arab Conquests* (United Kingdom: Hodder & Stoughton).

Haykal, Muhammad Husayn (1976): *The Life of Muhammad* (North American Islamic Trust: American Trust Publications).

Joiya, A. A., Hassan, R. S., & Joiya, A. Z. (2016): *Patient Satisfaction with Health Care Service Providers in Pakistan. A Review of Public Sector Hospitals of Lahore* (Germany: GRIN Publishing)

Kelen, Betty (1977): *Muhammad: The Messenger of God* (New York, Pocket Books).

Khan, S.A. (2016): *Governance in Pakistan: Hybridism, Political Instability, and Violence* (Pakistan: Oxford University Press).

Khan, Sara (2016): *'Retrieving the Equilibrium and Restoring Justice: Using Islam's Egalitarian Teachings to Reclaim Women's Rights'*, in *Sensible Religion*, (United Kingdom: Routledge).

Klainberg, Marilyn (2010): *'An Historical Overview of Nursing'*, in *Today's Nursing Leader: Managing, Succeeding, Excelling* (Unites States: Jones and Bartlett Learning).

Margoliouth, David Samuel (1939): *Mohammed* (London: Blackie & Son Ltd.).

Mernissi, F. (1991): *Women and Islam: An Historical and Theological Inquiry* (United States: South Asia Books).

Niaz, U. (2011): *Wars, Insurgencies, and Terrorist Attacks: A Psychosocial Perspective from the Muslim World* (Pakistan: Oxford University Press).

Nishtar, S. (2009): *Choked Pipes: Reforming Pakistan's Mixed Health System* (Oxford University Press).

Ordoni, Abu Muhammad (2014): *Fatima the Gracious* (Iran: Ansariyan Publications).

Patel, R. (2010): *Gender Equality and Women's Empowerment in Pakistan* (Pakistan: Oxford University Press).

Plowright, David (2011): *Using Mixed Methods: Frameworks for an Integrated Methodology* (California: Sage Publications).

Rahman, T. (2012): *The Class Structure of Pakistan* (Pakistan: Oxford University Press).

Razwy, Sayyid Ali Ashgar (2014): *A Restatement of the History of Islam and Muslims* (Lulu Press, Inc).

Renzetti, C. M., Edleson, J. L., & Bergen, R. K. (2001): *Sourcebook on Violence against Women* (USA: Sage).

Roberts, M., Hsiao, W., Berman, P., & Reich, M. (2003): *Getting Health Reform Right: A Guide to Improving Performance and Equity* (New York: Oxford University Press).

Robinson, F. (2000): *Islam and Muslim History in South Asia* (USA: Oxford University Press).

Saikia, Y. (2011): *Women, War, and the Making of Bangladesh: Remembering 1971* (USA: Duke University Press).

Sen, A. (2007): *Identity and Violence: The Illusion of Destiny* (Great Britain: Penguin Books).

Seneviratna, Anuradha (1995): *King A☐oka and Buddhism: Historical and Literary Studies* (Buddhist Publication Society).

Shaheed, F., & Shaheed, A. L. (2011): *Great Ancestors: Women Claiming Rights in Muslim Context* (Pakistan: Oxford University Press).

Shaheed, Farida, and Neelam Hussain, (2007): *Interrogating the Norms: Women Challenging Violence in an Adversarial State* (Sri Lanka: International Centre for Ethnic Studies).

Shariati, Ali (2014): *Fatima is Fatima* (Lulu Press, Inc).

Siddiqui, S. (2014): *Language, Gender and Power: The Politics of Representation and Hegemony in South Asia* (Pakistan: Oxford University Press).

Smith, Cecil Woodham (1951): *Florence Nightingale* (New York City: McGraw-Hill Book Company).

Spencer, Jenny S. (1989): *'Marsha Norman's She-tragedies', Making a Spectacle: Feminist Essays on Contemporary Women's Theatre*, ed. Lynda Hart (Ann Arbor: University of Michigan Press).

Valiathan, M.S. (2003): *The Legacy of Caraka* (India: Orient Blackswan).

Wilkinson, Alice (1958): *A Brief History of Nursing in India and Pakistan* (Delhi: Trained Nurses' Association of India).

Zaidi, S. A. (1988): *The Political Economy of Healthcare in Pakistan* (Pakistan: Vanguard Books).

# Index

241